Laboring Out of Life

Laboring Out of Life

A DEATH DOULA'S APPROACH TO INTENTIONAL END-OF-LIFE CARE

KACIE GIKONYO

JOSSEY-BASS™
A Wiley Brand

Published by John Wiley & Sons, Inc., Hoboken, New Jersey.

Library of Congress Cataloging-in-Publication Data is Available:

ISBN: 9781394355730 (Hardback)
ISBN: 9781394355754 (ePDF)
ISBN: 9781394355747 (ePub)

Cover Design: Paul McCarthy
Cover Art: Olga Siletskaya/Getty Images
Author Photo: Courtesy of the Author
SKY10162105_070826

For my boys,
Jon, David, and Jackson.

You are the reason I believe the world is worth changing.

Contents

A Letter to the Reader

Hi.

If you're holding this book, I already like you.

Seriously. You picked up a book about death. On purpose. That tells me a few things right away. You're curious. You're brave. And you're probably a little tired of everyone whispering around a topic that's coming for all of us anyway.

So, let's just name it from the start: this book is going to teach you some things. It's also probably going to make you cry. (Sorry. Occupational hazard. Side effect of being a death doula.) I might scare you a little in places. That's not because I'm dramatic. It's because death has a way of pulling the curtain back on things we usually avoid looking at too closely.

We're going to talk about death openly here. Honestly. Without euphemisms. Without sugar-coating. Without pretending it's something "beautiful" all the time or something we can slap a bow on to make it more comfortable. Sometimes death is peaceful. Sometimes it's messy. Sometimes it's sacred. Sometimes it's exhausting. Often, it's all those things in the same afternoon.

Buckle up.

This book is not here to sell you a fantasy version of death work or dying or grief. It's here to tell the truth. The kind of truth that actually helps. The kind that makes you feel steadier instead of more afraid. The kind that lets you say the word *death* out loud without lowering your voice.

You don't need to be a death doula to be here. You might be thinking about becoming one. You might already be doing this work. You might work in healthcare, hospice, funeral service, caregiving, or the grief world. You might just be death-curious and wondering why this topic keeps tugging at you. All of that is welcome here.

And if you are reading this because something in you is considering becoming a death doula, I want you to know there is a place for you in this work. I created Death Doula School for people just like you. People who feel the calling, even if they cannot fully explain it yet. People who want to support others through one of the most human experiences we will ever face.

If that is you, I would love to walk with you in a deeper way. You can learn more at deathdoulakacie.com or find me on social media @deathdoulakacie, where I share education, resources, and what this work actually looks like in real life.

Read this book at your own pace. Put it down when it gets heavy. Come back when you're ready. There's no gold star for powering through. Death has excellent timing and terrible manners, but this book will wait for you.

And before we go any further, let me say this clearly: I'm really glad you're here. I don't think people stumble into this work, or this topic, by accident. Something led you here. Curiosity. Loss. Calling. A quiet nudge you couldn't ignore. Whatever it was, you listened.

That matters.

So take a breath. Get comfortable. And let's talk about the thing no one wants to talk about but everyone needs to understand.

I'll walk with you.
—Kacie

Introduction

If you really want to understand how I ended up here, you have to start at the beginning. Not with nursing school or death work, but with the place where I first learned to feel completely at home with death, right down the road from my grandma's house: All Saints Cemetery.

It sounds strange, I know. Most kids were riding bikes, trading Pokémon cards, or doing whatever normal children did in the 90s. Meanwhile I was wandering through a cemetery like it was my own personal sanctuary. I wasn't being spooky or disrespectful. It was the opposite. I was just. . .home. The cemetery was the only place quiet enough for my brain to breathe, to think, to settle.

I'd walk the rows of headstones, fingertips trailing over cool granite, reading names out loud as if the universe might forget them otherwise. I invented whole lives for them. Who they were. Who they loved. Who loved them back.

My best friend would sometimes come with me, mostly against her will. She jumped at every squirrel and snapping twig while I lingered near the heart-shaped pond, searching for frogs like a cemetery-dwelling forest fairy, while she pleaded for us to leave.

I didn't have the language for it at the time, but looking back, I know why I loved it so much. It was the only place where life and death felt like they were part of the same story. Peaceful. Human. Honest. No one avoided the truth. Everything was out in the open.

And honestly? I think that's where this book really began.

Because somewhere along the way, the world forgot that death is human. We tucked it behind hospital curtains, medical jargon, and cultural fear. We turned it into something clinical, sterile, distant. A taboo. A secret. We transformed death from a fact into a failure.

Why do we accept deaths that feel rushed, sterile, and disconnected as inevitable? Why do we treat dying as something to get through instead of something to tend to?

That's the myth I'm here to smash wide open.

Death is not a dirty word.

Say it again if you need to. Louder this time.

You're holding this book because, whether you realize it or not, you're ready to look at death differently. Maybe you want to become a death doula. Maybe you work in healthcare and you're tired of feeling like the human side of dying keeps getting pushed to the bottom of the chart. Maybe you're grieving. Maybe you're not grieving yet but you want to understand what's coming someday. Maybe you're simply curious, the way I was as a kid wandering between gravestones trying to imagine the full stories of strangers.

Whoever you are, I know one thing for sure: you're here because you seek meaning. You want clarity. You want truth, not the watered-down version.

And you're in the right place.

This book is going to change something in you, not because I'm trying to be dramatic but because you simply can't sit with death this long without being changed. I'm not here to scare you. I'm not here to preach to you. I'm here to open a door and say, "Come on in. This room isn't as dark as you think."

I'll tell you the real stories, mine and my clients', the ones full of grit, beauty, humor, heartbreak, and humanity. I'll teach you the skills and tools I wish I'd had sooner. I'll show you what this work looks like from the inside. And if you decide along the way that you want to walk this path yourself, I'll show you how to do that too.

We'll dismantle the misconceptions one by one.
We'll untangle the fear.
We'll rebuild a truth that honors the human experience.

And by the time you reach the end of this book, I hope you'll do something that has changed my entire life:

Sit with your dying self for a moment each day.

Ask her what matters.
Ask her what doesn't.
Ask her what needs to change in your life right now, while you still have time to change it.

Because death isn't here to take from us. She's here to remind us what living really is.

So, take a breath. Settle in. Get comfortable.
You and I are about to walk through something big together, something honest, something human, something that's been waiting for you.

And I promise you this: by the end of this book, you won't look at death, or life, the same way again.

Now turn the page, Love.
We're just getting started.

PART I

The Work

CHAPTER 1

Death Work Is Life Work

After all those afternoons wandering All Saints Cemetery whispering names off headstones, I thought I understood something about death. I thought I had the vibe down: quiet, peaceful, earthy. I thought death would always feel like grass under my shoes, cool stone under my fingers, some mysterious hush that didn't need to be feared.

But nothing, I mean nothing, prepares you for the first time death shows up in front of you not carved in stone, not tucked neatly under the ground, but happening right there in a bed only a few feet away from where you're standing. Nothing prepares you for the moment death stops being a concept and becomes a person you've grown to care about.

I was a new nurse in a long-term-care facility, still figuring out where everything lived in the supply closet and how to clock in without messing it up. And like most new nurses, I had latched onto a couple of favorite residents right away. We're not supposed to have favorites. . .but we all do.

One of mine was a man with developmental disabilities who met me at the nurses' station every single morning. Every day. Same time. Same smile. He didn't have any living family, no visitors, no one calling to check on him. The staff was the only family he had left, and we loved him the way family loves you, with softness, with humor, with candy bars slipped into his hands when no one was looking.

That morning, the nurses station felt off before I even got my coat off. He wasn't there.

I felt it immediately, that weird internal shift when something is wrong and your body knows before your brain does. I asked where he was.

A co-worker shrugged and said, "He's actively dying."

That phrase meant nothing to me at the time. No one had taught me what "active dying" looks like or what it even means. It wasn't part of orientation. No one sat down and said, *Here's what happens to a human body when it's nearing the end, and here's how to support them.* I was learning by fire.

I went straight to his room. He was lying in bed, eyes open, terrified. Not uncomfortable, terrified. He kept saying he was scared. He kept calling out for help in this panicked, pleading voice, and my heart just dropped. I held his hand and tried to reassure him, but I was new and barely holding it together myself.

This wasn't the peaceful, gentle death I'd imagined. This wasn't the quiet cemetery from my childhood. This was raw fear.

I went to the seasoned nurse on staff and asked what to do. She told me, without even looking up from her charting, "Call hospice and keep it moving. You've got 42 other patients today."

Her tone wasn't cruel. It was. . .normal. It was the routine. It was the system.

I called hospice. In my mind, I pictured someone arriving to sit with him. Someone who would take his hand, lower their voice, be the calm presence he needed. But the hospice nurse, kind as she was, had a full schedule, too. She adjusted his medications, made recommendations, and had to leave for her next patient.

And so, it was just. . .us. A facility full of good people with no time.

The rest of that day, I skipped lunch and used every spare minute I had to sit beside him, even if it was just for 60 seconds at a time. I'd run meds down the hall and then slip back in. Chart for a moment and then slip back in. I held his hand and told him he wasn't alone even though, deep down, I knew he mostly was.

He died on the twelfth hour of my shift.

I wasn't in the room. I was down the hall doing CPR on another resident. The alarms were blaring, people yelling orders, gloves snapping, the whole chaotic ballet of healthcare, and, meanwhile, my sweet morning greeter took his last breath alone in the dark.

I remember standing in the hallway afterward, leaning against the wall, just. . .stunned. Heartbroken. Angry in a way I didn't have words for yet. Not angry at anyone in particular angry at the system that left no time for compassion. Angry that dying people had become tasks instead of humans. Angry that he had cried for help and the best we could offer him was "I'll be right back."

In that moment, I understood something nobody had ever taught me in nursing school:

> *We are failing people at the end of their lives. Not because we don't care, but because the system doesn't allow us to show it.*

I didn't have the language for it yet. I didn't know the word *doula*. I didn't know anything about holistic end-of-life support. I just knew something was broken, and I couldn't unsee it.

That experience became the crack that let all the light in. It pulled me into death work long before I even realized I was heading there.

Since then, I've sat beside hundreds of dying people. I've heard their last words, their regrets, their whispered truths. And over and over, the themes repeat:

> "I wish I hadn't worked so much."
>
> "I wish I'd let myself be happy."
>
> "I wish I'd said what I needed to say."

That's when it hit me, hard and permanently:

> **Death work isn't really about dying. It's about living.**

When you sit that close to the end, you stop pretending you have all the time in the world. You wake up. You start paying attention. You start feeling your life again, not sleepwalking through it.

Death has a way of slapping the nonsense right out of you.
What matters starts to matter more.
What doesn't matter drops away.

And that's why this work matters.
That's why *this book* matters.

Because when you accept that life is temporary, you finally start living on purpose.

The Misunderstanding of Death Work

Most people think death work is about dying. It's not.

When people hear "death doula," they picture someone sitting vigil, whispering final goodbyes, or lighting candles beside a body. They imagine grief and sorrow, maybe even something morbid or spooky. What they don't realize is that death work isn't about the end at all; it's about everything that leads up to it.

It's about how we live, how we love, how we let go.

In healthcare, we're taught that death is a failure. The language alone exposes the culture:
"Expired."
"Coded."
"We lost them."
"Body ready for transport."

We rush to clear the room, cover the body, reset the bed.
Efficiency over humanity.
Checklists over presence.
Silence filled with tasks because stillness feels like failure.

But that first death showed me something else entirely.

That man didn't need another medication adjustment.
He didn't need another order set.
He needed someone to look him in the eye and say, "You're not alone."

But the system had no place for that.

That's why death doulas exist.

It's not that healthcare workers don't care; they care deeply. It's that they're trapped in a model that treats *dying as a problem to fix instead of a process to honor*. Nurses, doctors, and aides were trained to fight death tooth and nail but not to walk beside it.

Death doulas exist because no one should die scared and alone. No one should be so busy keeping people alive that they forget to help them die well.

Death isn't only medical work. It's mostly human work.

And we've misunderstood that for far too long.

As doulas, our job isn't to save lives, it's to hold them. To create a sacred pause in a world that doesn't like to stop. To remind people that there's beauty even in the hardest goodbyes.

It's the art of staying when everyone else is rushing away.

When I say, "Death work is life work," this is what I mean. The closer you get to death, the more clearly you see life. The more you witness loss, the more fiercely you love.

We don't fix death.
We witness it.

We don't avoid grief.
We make space for it.

We don't run.
We stay.

And in the staying, we learn what it means to be fully, deeply human.

What Death Work Teaches Us About Living

Death work teaches you gratitude in its rawest, least-Instagrammable form. Not the cute "gratitude journal" kind, the gritty kind. The kind where you wake up, take a breath, stretch your legs under the blankets, and think, *Damn, I get another day? Another shot?*

Because when you sit at enough bedsides, when you've heard enough last breaths, enough final confessions, enough whispered regrets, you start to understand something most people spend their whole lives trying not to think about:

> None of this is guaranteed.
> Not tomorrow.
> Not the next hour.
> Not even the next minute.

And once you let that truth settle into your bones, you stop wasting your time pretending you're promised a "later." You stop saving joy for the weekend. You stop waiting for the "right moment" to rest or apologize or tell someone you love them. You stop filling your life with things that don't matter because you finally understand, in the deepest way, that your time *is* your life.

That kind of awareness changes everything about the way you show up in the world. You parent differently. You love differently. You listen differently. You stop talking just to fill the silence and start respecting stillness as its own kind of medicine. You learn that presence, real, honest, undistracted presence is the most powerful gift you can ever offer another human being.

Over and over, death has shown me that while it takes from us, the people we love, moments we weren't ready to lose, chapters we weren't done living, it also *reveals*. It reveals what mattered most. It reveals the people who were worth our time and the ones who never deserved our exhaustion. It reveals how much of our lives we spend chasing things that never deserved our energy. Death is the great truth teller. It doesn't just strip life away; it strips life *down*, leaving only what's real.

It reminds us that the goal was never to live forever.
The goal is to live *fully*.

That's the irony of being a death doula. The closer you get to death, the more alive you become. The more time you spend with people who are dying, the more you realize how much of life you've been sleepwalking through. You start savoring the slow mornings. You linger longer in hugs. You notice the way your kid's hair smells when they climb into your lap. You say *no* more often. You say yes more intentionally. You stop apologizing for wanting a life that feels good.

And slowly, quietly, beautifully, you realize something else:

> Death isn't the opposite of life; it's part of it.
> It's the mirror every one of us will face someday.
> When it finally turns toward you, the only question it will ask is:
>
> **What did you do with the time you had?**

WHY IT MATTERS/THE INVITATION INTO THE WORK

Death work matters because somewhere along the way, our culture forgot what dying really is. We've turned it into a medical emergency, a problem to be solved, a failure to be prevented. We've tucked death into back rooms and hushed conversations and sterile hallways that smell like antiseptic instead of love. We've sanitized grief, rushed funerals, and conditioned people to think death is something shameful or frightening, something we don't talk about until we're forced to.

And in all that avoidance, we've lost something essential.
When we avoid death, we avoid truth.
And when we avoid truth, we stop living honestly.

That is why this work matters.
Death doulas bring humanity back to dying, and with it, bring meaning back to living.

We remind people that love still exists in the last hours. That forgiveness is still possible, that reconciliation can still happen, that a person can take their final breath feeling held instead of abandoned. We show families that presence is the most powerful medicine, and that silence, when shared with intention, can be holy.

Every person deserves to die feeling seen and cared for. Every family deserves guidance through the storm. And every community deserves to remember how to show up for one another in times of loss, not with fear but with tenderness.

This is the work.
And this is where **you** come in.

When a death doula walks into a space, confident, compassionate, unafraid, the room shifts. Fear softens. Shoulders drop. People breathe again. They realize, often for the first time, "Oh. We're allowed to talk about this. We're allowed to feel this. We're allowed to do this differently."

That's how the narrative changes, one conversation at a time, one bedside at a time, one brave human willing to speak the truth out loud.

Right now, most people remember the death of a loved one through a lens of panic: chaotic rooms, unanswered questions, fear hanging in the air like a second oxygen. Everyone rushing, everyone scared, everyone guessing. It becomes a traumatic memory because no one ever taught them another way.

But with a death doula in the picture, the entire story unfolds differently.

Instead of chaos, there is calm.
Instead of confusion, there is clarity.
Instead of loneliness, there is presence.

Families remember the beauty of the death plan their loved one created. They remember how they honored final wishes with reverence. They remember the peace of knowing what to do, how to do it, and why it mattered. They remember feeling connected. Supported. Held.

They don't just remember the moment of death; they remember the way it *felt*.
The warmth.
The intimacy.
The sacredness.

That is the power of this work.
We cannot stop death, but we can change the way people experience it and that changes everything.

Being a death doula isn't just a role you play. It's a calling. It asks you to show up with your whole heart, your intuition, and your humanity intact. It asks you to be comfortable in the places others avoid. It asks you to witness the softest, scariest, most honest moments of a person's life and hold space for them exactly as they are.

You don't need to have all the answers.
You just need to be willing to be there.

If you're reading this book, you're here for a reason. Something in you already knows that this work is sacred. Something in you is ready to unlearn the fear and step closer to the truth. Something in you wants to be part of changing the way we die and in doing so, changing the way we live.

So here is my invitation to you:

> **Step closer.**
> Learn what it means to labor out of life with grace, dignity, and humanity.
> Let this work soften you where the world has hardened you.
> Let it strengthen you where grief has made you small.
> Let it rearrange you. Let it grow you. Let it wake you up.

Because when you commit to death work, you're not just helping people die, you're helping the living remember how to live.

And every time you do that, you're rewriting the story the world tells about death, one family, one bedside, one sacred goodbye at a time.

REFLECTION: SITTING WITH YOUR DYING SELF

Before you move into the next chapter, I want you to do something that might feel a little strange at first, but I promise you, it will change the way you move through this book, and maybe even the way you move through your life.

I want you to sit with your dying self.

Not in a morbid way, not in a fearful way, in a deeply human way. In a way that lets you meet the wisest, softest, most honest version of you.

Find a quiet place if you can. Put your phone somewhere it can't vibrate in your ear. Let the noise and the lists and the obligations fade to the edges. Take a breath long enough to feel your ribs move. Then take another.

Now imagine yourself at the very end of your life.
Old.
Wise.
Soft around the edges.
Someone who has lived, loved, grieved, rested, and risen more times than you can count.

Picture that version of you looking back at the person you are right now, the one holding this book, curious enough and brave enough to be here.

And ask her:

> **Would my dying self be at peace with how I'm spending my days?**
>
> Would she feel proud of the way I love, the way I rest, the way I show up in the world?
>
> Would she feel that I lived with intention. . .or that I kept waiting for "later," as if later was ever guaranteed?

Let whatever answers rise to the surface. Don't push them away. Don't tidy them up. Don't judge yourself for what comes up, judgment is useless in this practice. Honesty is everything.

Just listen.

Your dying self is the version of you who no longer cares about perfection, reputation, or productivity. She cares about meaning. She cares about peace. She cares about whether you lived your life in a way that felt true to you.

Once you've listened, make one small promise to her.
Not a dramatic vow.
Not a full-life overhaul.

Just *one small thing* you'll start doing differently today.

Maybe it's slowing down while you sip your morning coffee so you actually taste it.
Maybe it's deleting a commitment you don't want to keep.
Maybe it's calling someone you love before the thought drifts away.
Maybe it's finally giving yourself permission to rest without guilt.

Death work isn't something you only do for others. It's something you practice in yourself.
It's a way of living.
A way of paying attention.
A way of remembering what matters before it becomes a regret.

The way you live your own life will become your greatest teaching tool, not just for your clients, but for your children, your friends, and every person who learns from your presence. The work starts with you. It always has.

When you're ready, turn the page.
There's so much more to learn and so much more life to live.

CHAPTER 2

Redefining the Good Death

The Measure of a Good Death

When I worked as a nurse, the phrase "good death" got tossed around like it was something simple. A checkbox. A shift note. A quiet room where nurses could walk out without wiping tears or mascara. In healthcare, a "good death" basically meant this: it didn't disrupt the floor.

If the patient died quickly.
If the morphine kicked in fast.
If hospice came and did most of the heavy lifting.
If the family wasn't screaming, wailing, or begging for more time.
If no one pressed the call light right afterward.
If the body could be zipped, documented, and transferred without chaos.

That, in the medical world, was considered "good."

My colleagues would say things like:
"At least they went peacefully."
"That one was easy."
"Quiet room, thank God."

And when they said "easy," they didn't mean for the patient.
They meant *easy for us*.

No alarms.
No code brown and code blue at the same time.
No frantic phone calls.

No breakdowns in the hallway.
No families second-guessing every decision.
No staff being emotionally cracked open.

But here's the truth most people don't see:
Healthcare professionals aren't trained to help someone die.
We're trained to interrupt it. Delay it. Fight it.
Death is the enemy. The failure. The thing we're supposed to prevent at all costs.

So, when dying *actually* begins, when the body shifts, when the breath changes, when the veil thins, most clinicians instinctively pull back. This is not because they don't care because they weren't taught how to stay.

It is also because the system they work in quietly redirects the entire trajectory of care long before they even realize it's happening. The system shifts the goal long before the people inside it ever would. What begins as saving slowly turns into managing, medicating, and doing whatever' is possible within impossible constraints. It's not avoidance; it's survival inside a structure that gives no time for presence.

And when a patient finally dies, the system calls it a "good death" if it didn't rattle us too much.

But when I became a death doula, that definition shattered.

A good death isn't about how well the staff coped.
It's about how deeply the person was known.
How much agency they still had.
Whether they felt like themselves until the very end.

I've seen a person's favorite song calm their entire nervous system more effectively than Ativan ever could. I've watched a daughter's hand resting on her mother's blanket do more to quiet breathing than oxygen or morphine. I've seen a spouse crawl into bed one last time just to hold their person the way they'd held them since their twenties, and the room shifts. The air softens. The body settles.

Medicine can soothe symptoms.
But intimacy soothes the soul.

A good death, I learned, is less about managing decline and more about honoring a life as it closes. What they loved. What they feared. What they wanted. What made them *them*.

One client taught me that lesson the hardest way of all.

She was in her thirties, young, vibrant, lived in yoga pants, and believed deeply in holistic wellness. She didn't trust Western medicine. At all. When she was diagnosed with an aggressive form of breast cancer, she refused chemo, radiation, surgeries, and, later, even hospice.

She hired me for the last six months of her life.
I supported her through herbal teas, essential oils, guided meditation, homeopathy, acupuncture. I held her hand during energy work sessions. I helped her create a death plan that reflected her values.

But as the cancer advanced, so did her suffering.

Her parents and I begged her to consider medical interventions purely for comfort. She was in agony. But she said no. Every time. She believed in natural healing, even in dying, and she trusted her beliefs more than our fear.

It was excruciating to witness.
The nurse in me wanted to ease her pain.
The mother in me wanted to save her parents from watching their child suffer.
The human in me wanted one moment when she wasn't wincing through every breath.

But the doula in me knew my job wasn't to steer her away from her truth.
My job was to honor it.

So I sat with her. I loved her. I supported her.
And she died the way she chose, wrapped in the belief system she lived and breathed.

From the outside world, people would call it a terrible death.
Cruel.
Unnecessary.
Avoidable.
Painful.

But it was hers.
Her truth.
Her decision.
And there is a quiet peace in that, even when the road is hard.

That client taught me something I never forgot:

> **The myth of the good death is that it's supposed to look a certain way. Quiet. Tidy. Serene. Painless. Predictable.**

But death, like life, refuses to follow scripts.

Sometimes it's calm.
Sometimes it's messy.
Sometimes it's loud or chaotic or filled with contradictions.
Sometimes it's soft and warm and holy.
Sometimes it's confusing and tangled and deeply human.

And sometimes the most peaceful deaths are the ones that never look peaceful from the outside.

We talk a lot about what makes a "good death," but rarely do we ask whose definition we're using.

The medical system's idea of a good death?
The family's?
The religious community's?
Your own personal belief system?
Or, novel thought, the dying person's?

As a nurse, I saw how quickly the system takes over.
As a doula, I've seen how powerful it is when we hand that power back.

A good death isn't measured by how comfortable it was for the staff or how gentle it looked or how quickly we can tuck the body away.

A good death is measured by alignment.
By the truth of it.
By whether the person died the way they wanted, not the way everyone else told them they should.

Some people want a quiet room.
Some want a full house and loud music.
Some want prayers.
Some want jokes.
Some want their dog in bed with them.
Some want lavender diffusing.
Some want their favorite show playing in the background.
Some want to die in their home.
Some want to die in a hospital where they feel safe.

There is no one version.

There is only the version that belongs to them.

And when we honor that, when we hand the mic back to the dying person, when we listen instead of assume, when we support instead of steer, that's when the real "good death" happens.

Because it's not about perfect endings.

It's about truthful ones.

Whose Death Is It Anyway?

We like to pretend that dying is personal. That when the time comes, the person doing the dying will be the one calling the shots.

But the truth?

Most of the time, once someone gets sick, their autonomy starts slipping out of their hands faster than anyone realizes.

Suddenly everyone has an opinion.

The doctor.
The spouse.
The adult children.

The church.
The neighbor who once read an article.
Google.
The system.

And in that tidal wave of voices, the one voice that actually matters the dying person's—gets pushed to the background like an afterthought.

There's one client whose story still sits heavy on my chest.

She had lived through cancer four separate times. Four full battles. Four rounds of chemo, radiation, ports, scans, hair loss, nausea, fear, and sheer grit. She had done everything medicine asked of her. And she won, every time.

By the time I met her, she was older. Tired. Quiet in a way that didn't come from defeat but from deep knowing.

We sat together in her living room, candles lit, herbal tea steaming, the kind of soft music playing that only people who've been through hell enough times choose as background noise. She held her mug with both hands like she was keeping herself steady, and she said the words that lifted 10 pounds straight off her shoulders:

> "I don't want to do treatment again. I'm done. I want peace."

Her whole body softened.
Her face unwound.
She even laughed a little, a tiny, relieved breath, because she finally vocalized the truth.

She wanted hospice.
She wanted comfort.
She wanted to spend whatever time she had left being *herself*, not a medical project.

Later that day when her husband came home from work, she shared the news with him—almost excitedly.

Only problem—he wasn't excited. He wasn't on board at all. He told her no.

He told her she wasn't "allowed" to stop fighting.
That she'd do more chemo "until the end."
That choosing comfort was giving up.

So she did what so many women do: she swallowed her truth to protect someone else's emotions. And four weeks later, she died chemo-sick, exhausted, and robbed of the peaceful chapter she wanted.

That's what happens when we let other people define what dying should look like.

It stops being about the person living it and becomes about the comfort of the people watching.

Families cling to words like *fight* and *hope* because they can't bear the idea of "letting go." But hope isn't one-size-fits-all. Sometimes hope means a cure. And sometimes hope means a soft landing, a gentle goodbye, a final chapter written in calm instead of chaos.

I've had families tell me, "Don't tell Dad he's dying."

I'll be the first to tell you, I'm not built for sugar-coating.
I don't lie to anyone, let alone dying people.
The fear in those requests always belongs to the *living*, not the dying.

Most of the time, those dying already know.
They can feel it in their bones, in their breath, in the way time suddenly moves differently. Pretending otherwise doesn't protect them, it isolates them.

When you refuse to name death, you take away their chance to say goodbye on their own terms.

As a nurse, I saw what happens when silence takes over.
End-of-life planning gets avoided like it's contagious, and then families get blindsided with what I call the double whammy:

Whammy #1: Their loved one is declining fast.

Whammy #2: They have no idea what their loved one wanted.

So, they're forced to make impossible decisions in the middle of heartbreak, and no matter what they choose, someone ends up carrying guilt like a second skin. Wearing guilt and grief at the same time can be heavy.

As a death doula, my job is to prevent that from happening.

I help people complete their end-of-life paperwork, yes, but I also gather their families so everyone understands it. We talk through what matters most, what a meaningful death looks like to them, what they fear, what they want their final days to *feel* like. We build a death plan for not just the medical pieces, but the emotional, spiritual, and human ones too.

That's what autonomy looks like to me.

It's not control for control's sake.
It's dignity.
It's the right to decide how your own story ends, even if someone else doesn't like the ending.

And then, thankfully, there are the families who show us what support can look like.

Another client of mine battled cancer three different times throughout her long life. Despite this, she had lived a full, beautiful life. She had a career she adored, traveled often and everywhere, had a love story written in the stars. Her husband, the love of her life, had died five years earlier. By the time cancer returned again returned, she was in her late seventies. She didn't want more treatment. She didn't want to chase time. She wanted her final chapter to feel like *her*.

She told me this early on.
Clear. Calm. Certain.

She knew it, but she needed help telling her adult children, because that's a hard conversation no matter how old you are.

We planned it together, how she'd say it, what they might feel, how to hold the space.

And when she told them? They didn't fight her.
They didn't guilt her.
They didn't try to talk her into more suffering disguised as more time. They supported her with the kind of love that rearranges you.

Those children walked their mom home with grace. They honored every wish. They stood beside her like pillars. Watching them changed me as a mother. It reshaped how I talk to my kids about my own death, not to scare them, but to normalize it. To destigmatize it. To soften it. Because one day, they will face that chapter, and I want them to face it with clarity, not fear.

These stories, the hard ones and the hopeful ones taught me something important:
Every culture, every faith, every family system carries its own script for what dying "should" look like. And those scripts show up loudly at the bedside.

In some families, the oldest son automatically becomes the decision-maker even when he hasn't visited in months.
In others, religious communities insist on rituals or restrictions that overshadow comfort.
Some adult children can't handle the shift from child to caregiver, it's like trying to stand on legs you didn't know you had.
And spouses. . .usually the men. . .unravel like a loose thread the second things get real.

Then there are situations where comfort care gets tangled up with belief systems. I've seen families and even care teams lean harder on prayer or positivity than on actual symptom relief. Not out of cruelty, but because they're scared, overwhelmed, or following what they were taught to do in crisis.

But here's the uncomfortable truth:
Dying belongs to the person dying.
Everyone else is just a supporting role.

Our job as doulas, as families, as professionals is to help them write the ending *they* want, not the one we can most easily bear.

And once we honor that truth, we're ready to walk into the next part with open eyes.

Not the movie version of death, where everyone whispers and the lighting is excellent.
Not the sanitized version we tuck into eulogies.
But the real, unfiltered process of the body beginning its final work, the changes, the sounds, the shifts that make families panic and professionals scramble.

That part is sacred.
That part is human.
And that part is where real understanding begins.

The Reality of Dying

Death is not a single moment. It's not one dramatic exhale followed by a peaceful fade-to-black like every movie pretends. If dying worked the way Hollywood shows it, my job, my training, and honestly this whole book would be about one long sigh and a soft piano note.

But that's not how death works.
Not even close.

Most people don't die instantly. Dying is a process—a slow, structured, incredibly intelligent unwinding of systems that once worked together to keep a body alive. It's not a light switch being flipped. It's a dimmer gently turning down, click by click, until the room grows quiet.

For most people, this process lasts three to fourteen days. We call it the active dying phase. It's the body's last labor, the final transition, a labor out of life. Everything the body does in that window, every breath, every pause, every change in skin color or temperature is purposeful. It's not failure. It's not fear. It's the body conserving energy for the most important task it has left: letting go.

I've sat with this process hundreds of times. I've watched the skin shift toward that grayish, earthy tone. I've seen the muscles relax until the face looks like the skin is just setting on top of it, rather than attached. I've felt that unmistakable stillness that settles in the room, like the air itself knows something sacred is happening.

And yes, there is a smell.
People never talk about that.

When the body begins its final transition, there's this faint, metallic, earthy scent that rises. Not sweet. Not rotten. Just. . .ancient. Like wet soil after a storm mixed with warm pennies. Some people never notice it. Others (like me) pick it up early, long before anything visible changes. It's the scent of a body returning itself back to the earth it came from. The first time I smelled it, I second-guessed myself. The hundredth time, I trusted it. Now, it's one of the cues that tells me the veil is getting thin.

Then there's the breathing.

Toward the end, breathing becomes irregular, long pauses followed by a burst of shallow breaths. These pauses, called *apnea*, can stretch for seconds or even minutes. Families often panic, leaning over the bed whispering, "Is this it? Is this it?" But it's not panic, it's rhythm. The body is slowly untethering itself.

And then comes the sound that terrifies everyone: the death rattle.

If you've never heard it, it can shake you. It's a deep, rattling, gurgling sound caused by saliva and fluid pooling in the throat because the person no longer has the strength to swallow. It *sounds* like choking. It *sounds* like drowning. But it is neither.

The very first time I heard it as a baby nurse, I panicked too.
The family said, "It sounds like she's drowning!"
And in my head I said, "Yeah, it does!"

I had no idea what I was hearing. Nursing school hadn't covered real-world dying. So I did what any brand-new nurse does: I ran to get the seasoned nurse. She walked in, listened for half a second, and said, "Honey, that's normal," before explaining it in a way that calmed the family (and me).

Now, as a doula, I prepare people long before that moment ever arrives. When they understand what they're hearing—that it's not painful, not scary, just the body slowing down—the fear dissolves. Explaining how they can help can also give the family such relief during this time. A simple repositioning can help relieve the noise. Knowledge is power.

I once supported a family who'd learned from me months before. When the rattle began, they didn't panic. They didn't look at me with fear. They leaned in. They held hands. They whispered love instead of alarm. They knew exactly what to do, they helped to reposition their person and then they felt such relief that they knew what was going on, and how they could help. It was one of the most peaceful rooms I've ever stood in.

Not every family reacts that way, though.

I had a client deep in the active dying phase, surrounded by loved ones who had been diligently prepped by both hospice and me. But one family member, bless her heart, just could not accept what was happening. As soon as the breathing shifted, she panicked, called 911, and insisted on a hospital transfer. The ambulance ride was brutal on the patient's fragile body. By the time they reached the hospital, she died there instead of in her bed, surrounded by the family who loved her.

No shame.
No judgment.
Just grief acting out loud.

This is why understanding the physical process matters, because fear can rewrite an ending in seconds.

But then there are the moments that no textbook, no certification, no clinical training can explain.

My best friend Grace, who I've loved like a sister since childhood, lost her dad not long ago. I had known him my whole life. I stood beside her during his final hours. His breathing was shallow. His eyes were closed. His body had already softened into that almost-otherworldly stillness.

Grace squeezed his hand and asked me, "What do I do?"

I told her, "He can hear you. Tell him anything you want him to know."

So she leaned close and said, "Dad, I love you so much. It's okay for you to go."

And then, as if on cue, he opened his eyes.
Clear. Bright. Present.
He looked directly at her. The most intentional eye contact you've ever seen.

He didn't speak. He couldn't.
But that look said everything:

I love you too.

There was no fear in the room after that. Only love. Only release.

Moments like that are why I don't fear death. I've watched hundreds of people take their last breath, and not once has it felt like something dark or cruel. There is a shift, a softening, a lightening, and you can almost feel the soul move. It isn't an ending. It's a transition.

Energy doesn't die.
It changes form.
And witnessing that change over and over again has convinced me that whatever comes next isn't scary, it's simply the next part of the journey.

The reality of dying is messy and sacred, physical and spiritual, clinical and mystical all at once. It is not something to fix. It's something to accompany. Something to witness. Something to honor.

When we understand what dying looks like, the breathing patterns, the color changes, the stillness, the smell of the earth rising from the skin, we stop running from it. We stop fighting it. We stop misunderstanding it.

And when we stop misunderstanding death, we finally learn how to hold space for it.

Because understanding what happens to the body is only half the work. The other half is learning how to be the steady one in the room, grounded, soft, unafraid.

That's where a death doula becomes essential.
That's where this work becomes holy.

Redefining It for Ourselves

By now, you've probably realized there's no such thing as *the* good death.
There's no checklist.
No gold star.
No clean, crisp medical definition.

There is only *their* death, the one that belongs to the person doing the dying.

And when you've sat with as many people as I have, you learn quickly that what makes a "good death" isn't how it looks from the outside. It's how it feels from the inside. It's how deeply the person was honored in their final days, how fully their truth was allowed to exist without being overwritten by someone else's comfort, fear, or expectations.

I've seen deaths that most people would call "messy" turn out to be some of the most beautiful moments of a person's life. I've seen peaceful deaths that still carried an ache so deep it swallowed the room. I've sat in homes full of laughter, where kids were running through the hallway while someone was taking their last breaths and you know what? It was perfect. I've also sat in silent rooms where grief was so thick and sacred you didn't dare move too quickly.

And in every single one, there was meaning.
Not because it was tidy.
Not because it was serene.
But because it was true.

We've been taught to treat death like something that has to be hidden, sanitized, or prettied up, like grief won't hurt as much if we dim the lights and whisper. But when you step toward it instead of away from it, when you let it be what it is, the fear softens. It stops being the monster under the bed and becomes what it's always been: a human experience.

Redefining a good death starts with asking better questions.

Instead of:

> **"How do we make this easy?"**

We ask:

> **"What matters most?"**

Instead of:

> **"How do we keep them alive longer?"**

We ask:

> **"How do we help them live well until they're gone?"**

These questions change everything.

Whenever I sit with a client and ask them to imagine their ideal death, where they'd be, who they'd want there, what they'd want the room to feel like, they almost always cry. Not because they're scared, but because no one has ever asked them before. Their whole life, people have asked them about their career, their family, their plans, their dreams, even their retirement. . ..

But not their death.

And yet death is the only guaranteed chapter of the story.

So I ask:

Where do you want to die?
Who do you want in the room?
What do you want to smell?
What music do you want playing?
What would make you feel safe?
What do you want the people you love to remember when they think about your last moments on Earth?

These are not medical questions.
These are *identity* questions.
They're about meaning, comfort, belonging, legacy.

Sometimes people tell me they want to die outside under their favorite tree, the one whose roots feel like family. Sometimes they want candles (LED, because safety first!) and soft music. Sometimes they want their dog curled up beside them. Sometimes they want the whole house full, kids running around, dishes clattering, life spilling into every corner because that's how their life always was.

There is no wrong answer.
There is only the answer that belongs to *them*.
The only mistake is never asking.

As a doula, I've watched what happens when people get to shape their own ending. It unlocks a kind of peace you can't manufacture. A settling. A grounding. A sense of "okay, I know how I want this to go." I've also watched how planning their death helps people live more intentionally. The minute they stop pretending they're immortal, they start savoring everything, their morning coffee, their relationships, the ordinary magic they used to overlook.

That is the paradox of this work:

> *The closer you walk beside death, the more fiercely you understand life.*

A "good death" isn't just about dying well.
It's about living in a way that makes dying feel less like a theft and more like the next page of a story that was honest from beginning to end.

I once had a client, a retired teacher, who wanted to die surrounded by letters from her former students, boxes of handwritten notes from decades of children whose lives she shaped. Her family and I read them together as her energy faded. That was her good death. Not because it was painless or perfect, but because she felt complete.

Another client, a young mother, wanted the last thing she heard to be her children's laughter. She asked for her bed to be moved near the window, and on her final afternoon, her husband leaned down and said, "They're right outside." She smiled a soft, small, knowing smile and let go. That was her good death.

Different stories. Same truth:
A good death has nothing to do with perfection, and everything to do with presence.

What people want in death is the same thing they've always wanted in life:
To be seen.
To be heard.
To be loved.
To have some say in how their story ends.

If we can offer people autonomy, compassion, and understanding, we've already done something extraordinary.

When I sit with the dying, I often find myself wondering, *What would a good death look like for me?* It changes depending on the season of my life, but the core stays the same: peace, choice, connection, meaning. The same things I try to give every client.

That's what redefining a good death really is, reclaiming death as something deeply personal. Something sacred. Something human. Something ours.

When we stop chasing the myth of a "perfect" death and start honoring the personal one, death stops being a clinical event and becomes what it has always been:

A human experience.
A transition.
A continuation of the same love, truth, and presence that shaped a life.

And that is where the real work of death care begins.
Not in managing the body, but in meeting the soul.

CHAPTER 3

Navigating the Journey: Skills and Tools

The Heart of the Work

Death work begins long before you sit at a bedside.

It begins in the quiet space inside you, the part that knows how to pay attention, how to soften, how to stay.

By the end of Chapter 2, we talked about the soul of this work: presence, truth, meaning, connection. Now, in Chapter 3, we shift from what death *is* to what we actually *do* when we walk beside it. And before we talk about tools or techniques or anything remotely practical, we have to start here, at the center of the center, the heart of the work.

Because the best death doulas I have ever met weren't the ones with perfect résumés or endless credentials. They weren't the ones who could recite 10 stages of anything or quote obscure research studies. They were the ones with the biggest emotional range. They were the ones who felt deeply and didn't apologize for it. They were the ones who could walk into a room buzzing with fear and somehow become the calm.

The core of this work isn't technical skill. It's human skill.

Empathy.
Intuition.
Boundaries.
Listening without rushing to fix.
Being present without needing to perform.
Letting your heart stay open without letting it spill everywhere.

Empathy especially gets such an unfair reputation.
People tell me all the time, "I'm too sensitive for this work. I'd cry too much." And I always tell them, "That's exactly why you're perfect for it."

Empathy isn't fragility. It's a superpower.

It means you see more than the surface. You hear more than the words.
You notice the smallest shifts, the way a dying person keeps adjusting their blanket because they're cold, but they don't want to bother anyone. The way their son keeps stepping into the hallway pretending to be on his phone but is actually trying not to cry. The way the house feels, the way the air changes, the way grief breathes heavily even when no one has said a word.

Empathy is what keeps this work human.

And sensitivity?
Let me tell you something, this field would collapse without the sensitive ones. The world keeps telling sensitive people to "toughen up," but death work whispers, "No. . .soften. That's where your strength is."

But. . .empathy without boundaries will chew you up and spit you out.

I learned that the hard way.

Early in my death doula career, I poured myself into every family like I was the last drop in their emotional water bottle. I thought loving people meant giving them everything, my time, my energy, my mental space, sometimes at the cost of my own well-being. And guess what? That's the quickest route to burnout. Boundaries aren't about withholding love. They're about protecting your capacity *to* love.

They're not walls; they're anchors.
They keep you grounded so you don't drift into someone else's suffering and forget how to swim.

I used to think boundaries meant being cold, detached, or unavailable. But death work taught me the opposite. Boundaries made me softer. Kinder. Clearer. They gave me space to stay present instead of drowning in someone else's grief. They gave my clients the best version of me instead of the exhausted, overextended version.

And honestly, learning about boundaries changed everything about how I live my own life.

Before I became a death doula, I was working as an RN, with 12-hour shifts that magically turned into 16, rigid schedules that never budged, and a workplace that expected my *entire* life to orbit around my job. I wasn't overbooked because I couldn't say no. I was overbooked because the system didn't care whether I had kids, a family, appointments, or a functioning nervous system. I was constantly trying to wedge real-life doctor's appointments, choir concerts, and school events, even just breathing room into whatever scraps of time my work schedule didn't already own. I missed things, important things. I rushed everything. I stretched myself so thin I could see sunlight through my soul.

Becoming a doula flipped all of that on its head. My life comes first now, and my work fits *around* it. I don't miss the kids' events. I don't skip my own appointments. And sometimes I take a mental health day simply because I feel like it. Boundaries didn't shrink my world. They handed it back to me.

That's one of my favorite things about death work: when you spend your days sitting beside people who no longer have time, you get really clear about how you're spending yours.

Now, I protect my peace the way some people protect their retirement accounts.
If it drains me, it doesn't make the cut. If it costs me my peace, it's too damn expensive.

Watching people die teaches you, viscerally, that none of us gets to bargain for more time. Our time is now. Our life is the one we're living today, not the fantasy one we keep meaning to start next month.

Death work doesn't just teach you how to *do* this work; it teaches you how to *be*.

It teaches you to notice the way sunlight warms your kid's face in the morning.
It teaches you to savor your coffee instead of gulping it while rushing across the kitchen.
It teaches you that the people you love are on a time clock, too.
It teaches you presence—real presence, the kind that makes your whole life feel more intentional.

I tell my students all the time:

> **"Death work changes you at the cellular level."**

And it does.
You stop taking things for granted.
You stop performing your life and start living it.
You learn to love deeper and let go cleaner.

And the more you learn to live with your eyes wide open, the more natural every other death doula skill becomes.
Holding space.
Communicating clearly.
Maintaining boundaries with compassion.
Reading the room intuitively.
Showing up without needing to fix or control.

When you understand the heart of the work, really understand it, then everything else falls into place. And so the next question becomes:

How do we speak this work?

How do we communicate about death in ways that soothe instead of startle, comfort instead of confuse, open doors instead of shut them?

Because the heart of the work is one thing. But knowing how to *voice* it, how to talk about death with steadiness and grace and truth, that's the next essential skill. And that's where we go next.

Communication: The Real Medicine

If you'd asked me five years ago, when I was working as an RN, what the most powerful medicine at the end of life was, I would've told you it was morphine.

Now that I am a doula and an RN, I know it's communication (with morphine as a close second).

The way we speak, the tone we use, the energy behind our words—that's what shapes how people experience dying. Words become either a balm or a burden. They can calm a nervous system or send it spiraling. They can bring clarity or create confusion. They can make death feel like a monster or a moment.

And the biggest mistake I see new doulas and even seasoned healthcare workers make is being afraid to talk about death. They tiptoe around it like it's an unstable floorboard. They whisper. They tighten their jaw. They look at the floor when they say the word dying, or worse, they don't say it at all.

They hide behind soft phrases like "passed away" or "gone on" or "they're comfortable now." They use poetic language because they think it's gentler, but all it really does is make people feel like they're not getting the full truth.

But here's the thing: the discomfort doesn't come from those dying. It comes from *us*.

We project our fear, our uncertainty, our own unresolved feelings about death into the room, and the people around us mirror it right back. Humans are emotional tuning forks. If you talk about death with dread, they'll feel dread. If you talk about it calmly, compassionately, directly, they'll match that steadiness.

That's why I tell my students all the time:

> **You set the tone. If you stay calm, they'll stay calm. You are the nervous system of the room.**

You can say the most accurate, helpful, medically correct sentence in the world, but if your energy is shaky, it will land shaky. I have *never once* had someone respond negatively to me when I've spoken clearly and compassionately about dying. Not one single time. The secret isn't in the words; it's in the way we say them.

Real communication in death work isn't about memorizing a script, though you know your girl loves a good script. But communication is alive. It's relational. It shifts with the room.

It's about learning to show up with honesty and humanity.
It's knowing when to speak, when to pause, and when silence is the medicine.
Most people listen just to respond.
Death doulas listen to understand.

That's what active listening really is: being present enough to hear what's underneath the words. Hearing the tremble in a spouse's voice when they say, "We're okay." Noticing the adult child pacing in the hallway because they're trying not to fall apart in the room. Seeing what's happening even when no one is naming it.

Holding space isn't about having the answers. It's about creating a container big enough for whatever shows up—fear, grief, confusion, panic, regret, love—and meeting it with complete nonjudgment.

I once had a client in his late fifties with aggressive brain cancer. A genius, truly one of those freakishly smart people whose brain seemed to run 10 steps faster than the rest of us. He built airplane engines for Boeing. Built them. Until one day, he couldn't remember simple things. Then he struggled to speak. Then came the scans: tumors everywhere. Tumors no surgeon could remove without destroying the very things that made him *him*.

His sister was his caregiver. His elderly parents were still alive. And they were desperate, sweetly, heartbreakingly desperate. They tried everything: vitamin infusions, pills, diets, research studies that made absolutely zero clinical sense. Anything that offered even the faintest whiff of hope.

But with brain cancer like his, every day brought something new that he lost. Sight in one eye. Movement in his arm. Speech. Continence. And once he lost something, it *never* came back.

After months of trying everything, I could see it in his eyes. . .pain. Not physical pain, but the emotional weight of losing himself piece by piece. I've worked with a lot of dying people, and there is a particular look someone gets when they're ready. A kind of surrender that isn't giving up, it's acceptance.

So one day, with his family there, I sat next to him and asked gently, "Are you tired of fighting?" He could only nod yes or no. He nodded yes.

Then I said, "Do you want us to stop trying to save you and just focus on keeping you comfortable as you labor out of life?" He nodded again.

The entire room shifted. It was like all the air settled.
Like everyone finally saw what I had been seeing in his eyes. The chaos softened. The frantic searching for something to fix calmed. The grief didn't disappear, but it transformed into something quieter. Something honest.

He died two weeks later, peaceful. Calm. Comfortable.
His family thanked me over and over, because they had been so busy fighting that they forgot to ask him what he wanted. They didn't know how to have that conversation.

That's what communication does.
It opens a door that people don't know how to open on their own.

Before I was a doula, I worked in long-term care. You'd think that in long-term care, where death is as common as blood pressure checks, that everyone would be comfortable with it. But some nurses were terrified. Some avoided dying patients altogether. Some refused to give morphine because they didn't "want to be the one who killed them." Some avoided calling hospice because they sincerely believed hospice killed people.

The worst communication failures were always the same:

The avoidance of naming what was happening.

I once watched a nurse walk into a family meeting and say, "Well, things are changing. They're slowing down. They're. . .you know. . .." And then she waved her hand around like she was shooing away a fly.

The family was confused and panicked.
"What does that mean?" they asked.
"Is she dying?"
The nurse just said, "Well. . .she's declining."

Declining.
In the moment they needed clarity, she gave them a crossword clue.

The family spiraled, thinking she might "bounce back" or that maybe she just needed fluids or that there was something they were missing. That nurse didn't mean harm; she was afraid. But her avoidance left the family unprepared, unsure, and more anxious than they needed to be.

And standing there watching it, I remember thinking:

This is why death doulas exist.

Not to replace healthcare. But to bring humanity back into it.

People say wild things at bedsides. I once had a son sit beside his dying father, squeeze his hand, and say, "Dad. . .the Browns today. So if you were thinking about heading out, honestly? This might be your moment." It was absurd and tender and so deeply human that I had to stare very hard at the wall to keep myself together. People cope in strange ways, and sometimes humor is the only thing keeping them upright.

Tone matters. Delivery matters. Intent matters most.

So many people assume that when someone stops speaking, stops responding, or keeps their eyes closed, they're "gone." But that's not true.

I've had clients who were in such deep end-of-life sleep that it seemed as if they weren't aware at all, until I said something cheeky and they gave me a tiny half-smile.

I had one woman who was tense, uncomfortable, waiting for medication to kick in. Her family was distraught. I put on her favorite music, The Beatles, and within seconds, her whole body softened. A little smile touched her lips. Her breath slowed. She melted into the sound.

These moments remind me every single time:
They're still here. They hear us. They feel us. They know.

Connection doesn't end when speech does. It just shifts to a quieter channel.

I said it before, but it's important so I will say it again. Remember:

> **If you stay calm, they'll stay calm. You are the nervous system of the room.**

Your tone regulates the space. Your presence sets the pace. Your steadiness becomes their steadiness.

Communication is safety.
Communication is clarity.
Communication is dignity.

Good communication at the end of life isn't about perfect words; it's about presence, intention, and energy. It's about reminding people, living and dying, that they are safe, seen, and not alone. When we can do that, when we can speak with truth and tenderness, we turn our words into medicine.

Now, as powerful as communication is, there are moments when even words fall short.

Moments when what's needed isn't another sentence but a deep breath. A steady hand. A quiet presence.

And that's where we go next:

> **Learning to hold space when it's hard.**

Anyone can be calm when everything's calm.
The real skill, the real test of a death doula, comes when the room is spinning. When grief gets loud. When anger flares. When tension is

so thick you can feel it sitting on your skin. That's when holding space becomes everything.

People often think holding space means doing nothing. But that's not even close to true.

Holding space is an *active* kind of stillness. A deliberate softness. A conscious decision to stay steady when the emotional weather in the room is torrential.

It means you choose not to fix, not to manage, not to perform, not to make the pain disappear.
You become the steady heartbeat in the middle of the chaos.
You ground the room just by being there.

At the end of life, what most people crave isn't advice.
It isn't solutions.
It isn't "the right words."
It's presence.

I've lost count of how many dying people have said to me, "I just need someone here."
Not talking.
Not rushing.
Not distracting themselves with tasks or pretending to be busy.
Just here.

That's the gift of holding space: being the person someone can trust to *stay*.

I remember a woman who was actively dying and wanted peace more than anything. She had made that clear. She wanted quiet. She wanted calm. She wanted to rest.

Her family, however, had other plans.

Within minutes of arriving at her bedside, they started arguing, not about her, not about anything that actually mattered, but about each other. Old wounds. Old grudges. Money. Family politics that should've died decades earlier. The room filled with noise, and I watched her trying to rest in the middle of it, her breath shallow, her brow tight with discomfort.

That was the moment I stepped in.

I didn't raise my voice, and I didn't scold them.
I just spoke softly and said, "She made it clear she wants calm. If you can't bring calm into this room, I'm going to have to ask you to step out so she can have what she asked for."

Silence.
The kind that makes your pulse thump in your ears.

And then. . .they left.

The energy shifted immediately.
The noise left with them.
I stayed by her side, holding her hand, breathing slowly, regulating the room with my body more than my words.
Her shoulders dropped.
Her face softened.
Her breath found a gentler rhythm.

She let go in peace.

That's holding space.
It's not passive.
It's not weak.
It's fierce compassion.
It's protecting peace like it's sacred, because it is.

But holding space doesn't always look like quieting a chaotic room. Sometimes it looks like sitting in the middle of heartbreak and not moving an inch.

I once worked with a family losing the matriarch, a woman in her fifties, a planner to the very end. She had two daughters in their early twenties and a husband who adored her. She planned every detail of her death, not because she was morbid but because she wanted to leave her family as prepared as humanly possible. She even hired, in her words, "the best death doula money can buy!"
(She said it, not me.)

Her biggest goal was to make it to her oldest daughter's wedding.
Six months away.

If I'm being honest, I didn't think she'd make it.
Neither did her hospice team.
But we prepared for that wedding like it was life itself, outfits, energy pacing, transportation, comfort plans, contingencies.
We held hope without lying about reality.

And then, against every medical expectation, she made it to that wedding.

And she didn't just attend that wedding.
She *thrived.*

She danced with her daughters.
She saw all her people.
She glowed in every photo.
For a day, she was her old self again.

The day after, the family was euphoric.
They were convinced this meant she was turning a corner, that healing was coming, that maybe, just maybe, she was getting better.

But she wasn't.

The wedding was her rally, her last great gift to her girls, her husband, herself.

She died three days later.

Her daughters shattered.
They cried.
They yelled.
They sat silent.
They fell apart and came back together and fell apart again.

And I held space for all of it.

I sat with them for hours, letting their grief move however it needed to move.
Anger.
Fear.
Confusion.

Guilt.
Memories.
Silence thick enough to feel like a blanket.

I didn't try to fix their grief.
I sat inside it with them until it softened enough to breathe around.

Eventually, once the first tidal wave settled, we were able to look up from the debris and see the sun through the clouds, the profound beauty of what she accomplished.
She made it to that wedding.
She danced.
She celebrated her daughter's marriage *and* the fullness of her own life in the same breath.
And her family had given her the exact moment she had been living for.
There is grief in that, yes.
But there is awe, too.

This is holding space.
It's letting grief be what it is.
It's letting love take the shape it needs to take.
It's letting people crack open without trying to glue them back together.

And here's the hardest part of all: you cannot hold space effectively if you're carrying everyone else's energy inside your own body.

Families project fear, guilt, unresolved trauma, old family dynamics, panic.
If you absorb it, you'll drown in it.
And if you drown in it, you cannot be the calm in the storm.

I've learned to pay attention to my own nervous system.
When I feel myself buzzing, tightening, bracing, I pause.
I use box breathing, four counts in, four counts hold, four counts out, four counts hold again.
It pulls me back into my body.
It reminds me I am not here to fix anything.
I am here to *be*.

Sometimes I close my eyes for two seconds and bring myself to the quiet patch of nature I always return to in my mind—the sun on my face, the sound of wind moving through leaves, the world continuing gently around me.
It grounds me every time.

Holding space is matching the rhythm of nature.
Steady.
Unhurried.
Unshakable.

You don't stop the storm.
You become the calm in it.

And once you learn how to hold space for others, the next step is understanding the practical side of the work, the tools, rituals, and simple items that support comfort and connection at the bedside.

That's where we go next.

Tools of the Trade

When people picture a death doula, they sometimes imagine someone showing up with incense and a drum, chanting softly in a dimly lit room. And sure, sometimes there's incense and chanting. I'm not completely opposed to a good chant. But most of the time, there's also a notebook, my favorite pen, a Bluetooth speaker, and a bag full of things that make the final days more comfortable, more personal, and more human.

There's no one-size-fits-all toolkit in this work. Every client has different needs, different comfort items, different histories, different energies. So my bag looks a little different every time I pack it. But there are a few things that are always inside, my fundamentals, the things that keep me grounded and prepared for whatever a day might bring.

There are the practical tools:

- Sponge swabs for mouth care
- My notebook and pen for documenting symptoms and conversations

- A small speaker for music or guided relaxation
- A pulse ox to monitor the rhythm of the body's shifting patterns (the nurse in me needs this one)
- Hustle Butter, a natural, lightly scented balm I swear by for hand massages

And then there are the emotional tools in the bag, the ones that technically aren't tools but absolutely function as such. A soft scarf I've had for years that I unconsciously reach for when I need grounding. A specific pen that has traveled through countless vigils. A tiny plant propagation, because I'm a plant mom with more greenery in my home than any reasonable human needs. I propagate my plants constantly, and when I go to a family's home, I often bring a baby plant with me. Something alive. Something growing. A quiet reminder that life continues, even in the presence of death.

These things may sound small, but they're steadying. They anchor me, and in turn, they anchor the space.

Then there are the "sometimes" items, the ones that depend entirely on the person I'm caring for. Some clients love essential oils. Some adore hand massages and request them every visit. Some find peppermint comforting; others prefer lavender. And sometimes, there are kids in the home, kids who don't quite understand what's happening, but intuitively sense the heaviness in the air. I keep coloring books and a few small pieces of candy in my bag for them. These little moments of normalcy matter. Children deserve a compassionate space to process, too.

And then there's the most important tool of all: the binder. I create one for every single person I work with, and it becomes the heartbeat of their care. It doesn't live in my bag; it lives right by their bedside, and inside it is everything we might need:

- End-of-life paperwork
- Their personalized death plan
- Hospice contacts, emergency numbers, and quick-reference info
- Important family phone numbers
- Notes about comfort routines, spiritual or cultural rituals, and emotional needs

- Space for legacy letters, obituary drafts, or messages to those they love
- Passwords or secure access instructions for phones, computers, and essential online accounts
- Instructions for social media, subscriptions, and cloud storage

When emotions run high, and they always do, families lose the capacity to remember details. They can't remember names or numbers or where they set down the paperwork the hospice nurse gave them two weeks ago. But the binder? It's the steady anchor in the chaos. Something solid. Something organized. Something that says, "Here's what you need. You're not alone in this."

But tools aren't just the items we bring.
The space itself is a tool.
And in my work, shaping the space is one of the most important things I do.

Most people don't actively think about the environment they're dying in. They're too overwhelmed, too tired, too emotionally saturated. That's where I come in. Together with their family, we create what we call the "hospice room," the space where someone spends their final weeks, days, and moments.

This process can be surprisingly tender and surprisingly practical.

We start with decluttering.
Medical equipment has a way of taking over a room, turning it into a mini hospital. There's a time and place for equipment, of course, but too much of it makes the space feel clinical instead of comforting. So we clear out anything that's not serving the person anymore.

Sometimes, we paint the walls a new color.
A soft blue, a warm white, something that feels calm and restful. It's amazing how much a paint color can change the emotional temperature of a room. I've seen people visibly relax after a wall color changes from beige to a soothing, nature-inspired shade.

Then we decorate.
Photos of the people they love.

Images of the ocean if that's their happy place.
Horses, books, quilts, the things that make them feel like themselves.

A good hospice room doesn't look like a hospital room.
It looks like a person's life, gathered into one intimate place.

One client of mine wanted her final space to feel like her childhood beach vacations, the ones where she and her siblings would collect seashells until their buckets overflowed. So we transformed her room into a gentle coastal haven. We played ocean sounds softly on a speaker. We placed seashells along the windowsill. We lit an ocean-scented candle (the safe kind—no actual flames). Her family told me later that when they entered the room, it felt like exhaling. It felt like her. And that's the point.

And then there are the rituals, another kind of tool altogether.

Not every ritual is religious. In fact, many are not. Rituals are simply meaning-makers. They are moments of intentionality that give structure to the emotional landscape of the end of life.

One of my clients had a daughter who performed in theater. Every day, the mother requested one ritual: her daughter should sing to her. "Any song," she said. "As long as it's you." And so every afternoon, her daughter came into the room, sat beside the bed, and sang something, sometimes a musical number, sometimes something silly, sometimes a lullaby. It didn't matter what it was. It mattered that it was *her*. It was the bright spot of her day, the thread connecting them as she drifted further and further away from this world. That song was a tool just as much as the binder or the lotion or the swab sticks. It comforted her. It grounded her. It reminded her who she loved.

There was one client whose memory lives in my body to this day. She was holistic and deeply connected to natural comfort. Hospice offered her every appropriate medication, but she wanted something gentler, something that felt like *her*. One day, almost instinctively, I warmed a little Vicks between my palms and rubbed it onto the places where she carried pain, her back, her hips, her knees, her neck. Slow circles, steady pressure, intentional touch.

She closed her eyes and sighed, a deep release I hadn't heard from her in weeks.
"Better than morphine," she whispered.

(It wasn't. But that didn't matter. What mattered was that she felt cared for.)

It became our ritual.
Every visit.
Every day.
The open jar of Vicks waiting on her nightstand like a tiny blue companion.
I'd warm the ointment in my hands until the scent rose between us, and she'd relax the moment I touched her skin. Not because of the ingredients, but because of the care. Because rituals are their own kind of medicine.

As she continued to decline and enter into her last days of life, she couldn't speak much anymore. Her breaths were thin and scattered. One day I was rubbing her back, just like always, when she reached for my hand. Her fingers barely had strength, but the intention was unmistakable. She looked at me with heavy eyes and whispered, with everything she had left: "How does anyone ever do this without you?"

I smirked and told her to save her energy. She managed to whisper one last sentence, "Everyone needs a Kacie when they're dying." That ended up being the last thing she ever said to me.

She died a few hours later, peaceful, comfortable, and held.
The jar of Vicks stayed open on her nightstand, like it knew its job was finished too.

I have carried her words with me ever since.
They are the reason I teach. The reason I fight for this field.
The reason I believe, with my whole chest, that no one should have to die without a doula by their side.

Tools aren't props. They're not checklists. They're not things you use to "perform" death work. Tools are invitations: to connect. to comfort. to be present.

When someone is dying, their world gets very small.
They can't always leave their bed.
They can't always move their body.
Their senses shift.
Their energy drains.
Their autonomy narrows.

Tools widen their world again. Even if it's just by an inch.

A soft blanket reminds them they still deserve warmth.
A playlist reminds them they're still allowed joy.
A plant clipping reminds them life continues in quiet ways.
A binder reminds them that their wishes matter.

Tools create structure where everything feels unstructured. They create comfort where everything feels uncertain. They create connection where words fail.

And sometimes, a tool is simply silence.
Silence that tells the room: "I'm here. I'm not afraid. You're safe."

When I teach my students about tools, I tell them this: Don't get hung up on having the "right" ones. The right tool is the one that meets the need in front of you.

Maybe it's a sponge stick.
Maybe it's peppermint oil.
Maybe it's your calm voice.
Maybe it's a blanket.
Maybe it's Vicks.
Maybe it's a child's coloring book.
Maybe it's a song sung by a daughter to her mother.

And sometimes. . .sometimes. . .it's just you.

Your presence. Your steadiness. Your breath. Your willingness to sit there and hold the moment without rushing it, fixing it, or running from it.

That is the tool no one can teach you to pack. But it's the one that matters most.

The Inner Toolkit

Everything I bring into a vigil is practical: a speaker, mouth-care tools, lotion for hand massages, the little comfort items that make the room feel softer. But none of it works unless *I'm* steady. The real tools of this job aren't in my bag. They're inside me: my nervous system, my boundaries, my energy, my ability to stay calm when the room is anything but.

Death work will test every single one of them.
You will sit in rooms that vibrate with grief and exhaustion.
You will answer questions no one wants to ask.
You will watch people break open in ways they've held back for decades.

And if you don't know how to empty yourself afterward, how to separate what belongs to you from what belongs to them, you'll start to carry those rooms inside your body. That's why every death doula needs an inner toolkit, a set of practices that keep you grounded, clear, present, and able to return to your own life when you walk out the door.

BREATH

For me, it always starts with breath.
When the room feels thick with emotion, when someone's fear spikes the air pressure, when grief ripples through a family like electricity, I match my breathing to something slow and steady. Four counts in. Four hold. Four out. Four hold.
Box breathing: Four counts in. Four hold. Four out. Four hold.

It's simple. It's free. And it works every damn time. It brings my nervous system back into my body so I can lead with clarity instead of emotion. But breath alone isn't enough.

ENERGETIC HYGIENE

Over the years, I've learned how to practice what I call *energetic hygiene*. Before I walk into a client's home, I pause at the door and take a deep breath. I picture myself leaving my own worries outside, the grocery list, the kids' schedules, the laundry mountain threatening to avalanche. When I leave, I do the opposite. I imagine handing back everything that belongs to them. Their grief, their fear, their questions, their anticipatory loss. Not because I don't love them, but because carrying their suffering home doesn't help them. . .and it destroys me.

It's my way of not mixing my life with their death. And sometimes, your inner toolkit gets tested right in the moment, when you least expect it.

I once worked with a woman who was considering ending treatment and shifting her focus to comfort and living fully with the time she had left. She wanted clarity. She wanted honesty. She wanted a space where she could say the truth out loud without being shut down or guilted.

We talked through her wishes, gently, intentionally. She spoke about exhaustion. About wanting quality, not quantity. About not wanting to spend the rest of her days fighting for more days.

Her husband wasn't in the room at first.
But near the end of our conversation, he walked in and asked what we were talking about.

She told him plainly, bravely, "I'm entertaining the idea of stopping treatment."

And that was it, the moment the air snapped.

I watched anger flood his face. His eyes hardened. His voice rose like a slammed door.
"This is exactly why I didn't want to hire a stupid death doula! I knew this would happen! I knew she'd push you into doing things you don't want to do!"

His words hit the room like gravel thrown against glass, loud, sharp, chaotic.
He wasn't really angry at me. He was terrified.
He was grieving a future he hadn't been ready to face.
But fear doesn't come out neatly. It comes out sideways.

I could feel the heat in my own chest, the instinct to defend myself. That's the old version of me, the one from my early nursing years, the one who didn't yet know how to separate other people's pain from my own. The one who would have matched anger with anger.

But death work has changed me. My inner toolkit kicked in before my mouth did.
Breathe. Ground. Stay.
This isn't about you. This is about him trying not to drown.

I stayed steady. I didn't flinch. I didn't fold. I held space for his rage without absorbing it. And once the storm in him had cracked open enough to let air in, I gently facilitated a conversation between the three of us.

His wife looked at him, soft but firm, and said, "These are my wishes. They're not hers. *She* is the one who finally listened to me without getting explosive."

And then she added, "That's why I wanted a death doula."

Everything shifted after that. Not because I fixed it, but because I stayed steady long enough for them to find each other again. That's the inner toolkit in action.

You don't discover inner tools in the middle of a crisis. They're built on all the boring, ordinary days so they're there when the crisis hits. If you only practice grounding when someone is yelling, your body won't trust it. You have to train your nervous system to know, "This is what we do. This is how we come back to ourselves."

After visits like that one, my body feels it. Even if I stayed calm in the room, I can feel the echo of it—the raised voices, the fear, the grief that had nowhere else to go. If I don't do something with all of that, it just sits in me. It turns into tight shoulders, a clenched jaw, snapping at my kids, staring at my phone but not really seeing anything.

NATURE

One of my go-to resets is nature. When a death or a visit hits me hard, and yes, even seasoned doulas get hit hard, I go outside. No phone. No podcasts. No inspirational quotes. Just me and the world being itself. I walk. I breathe. The trees don't need anything from me. The wind lets me be messy. The sunlight reminds me the world is still turning, even when someone's story just ended. Nature is the only place where I never feel like I have to be "on."

And when that's not enough?

I get in my car, blast early 2000s Lil Wayne, and rap every word like he personally invited me onstage. Nothing resets my nervous system like a one-woman hip-hop concert in the front seat of my SUV. That's part of the inner toolkit too, doing whatever pulls you back into your own body after you've been carrying everyone else's pain.

Over time, I've outgrown some of my old coping mechanisms, too. In my early career, I used to numb myself with work. If things felt heavy, I'd take on more clients, more shifts, more responsibility, anything to avoid feeling my feelings.
Now? I'm a big advocate for feeling your feelings.
I don't shove them down anymore. I let them move.
I don't break open from pressure anymore; I release in real time.

And then there's the ritual I don't talk about often: I speak to my people after they die.

I tell every client, half joking but half not, "If you're able to come back and visit me after you make your transition, you better do it." And I believe, wholeheartedly, that the soul stays close for a little while after death. So, in the days following, I talk to them out loud. If something reminds me of them, I talk to the empty air like they're still here. Maybe they hear me. Maybe they don't. But it helps. It closes the space gently instead of abruptly.

Death doulas need closure rituals. Not just for clients, for us.

Sit in your car for a minute and breathe. Have a mini concert if it feels good. Wash your hands with intention. Whisper thank you. Cry if you need to. This is how we keep compassion from turning into burnout. And finally, the last tool, and the one most doulas forget to value. . .

COMMUNITY

This work can feel isolating if you try to hold it alone. You need people who understand the weight of what you carry, the ones who won't flinch when you casually mention the word "dying" over brunch, the ones who can hear the heaviness in your voice and respond with, "Tell me everything."

For me, that's the Death Doula Collective, a community of doulas from across the country who hold each other up, talk each other through hard cases, and remind one another that we are human, too. They have carried me through tough clients, overwhelming seasons, and moments where my own life felt like too much to hold alongside someone else's death. That group is invaluable to me. We don't just teach each other. We save each other.

The outer tools help others find peace. The inner tools help you keep yours.

When we learn to tend both, we stop simply surviving the work and start being shaped by it, in the best possible way. Being a death doula isn't about learning to face death. It's about learning to stay alive in the middle of it. And once we've gathered our inner and outer tools, we're ready for the next chapter: putting them into practice and guiding others through the full journey, start to finish.

CHAPTER 4

Who We Serve

The Person at the Center

The first time I meet a new client, my goal is simple: connection. Not a sales pitch. Not a performance. Not a monologue about what a doula does. Connection. Before anything else, that's what matters. And if that first meeting feels like friction or forced politeness, I trust that feeling. I don't try to bulldoze it. This work is too intimate to ignore intuition.

That initial consultation isn't just about them deciding if I'm the right fit for them. It's also about me deciding if they are the right fit for me. I know that sounds blunt, but it's true. I cannot give my whole heart and nervous system to someone who feels like the wrong energy match. And they shouldn't give theirs to me if I don't feel like a fit either. A mutual choosing happens here, and it's part of the sacredness of the work.

When I sit down with a potential client, I'm doing three things at once.

- I'm making them comfortable.
- I'm reading the emotional temperature of the room.
- And I'm quietly watching how the family moves around them.

Are they protective? Overbearing? Detached? Loving but anxious? Circling like guardian angels? Hovering like helicopters?

I pay attention to the family because it shows me the landscape I'm walking into. Where there is love, where there is fear, where there are old wounds. But the person at the center? They tell me who they are through their own words, their own choices, their own tiny details. That is where the real work begins.

The dying person isn't just dying. They are dying inside a family story, a marriage, a childhood, a culture, a history. Every home I enter is its own ecosystem.

I always encourage loved ones to be present for the first meeting, because they're usually the most apprehensive. They picture me walking in with incense and a tambourine, or worse, they whisper that I'm there to "speed things up." They're scared, and they don't know what a doula is.

So, I sit down on the couch or bedside, and I say something simple like, "My goal here is not to take anything away. My goal is to make this easier."

When they learn I'm not there to take over, the whole room exhales. I'm not trying to be their nurse or their doctor. I'm not speeding anything up. I'm not slowing anything down. I'm just here to make this experience kinder, calmer, and more human. I support the person dying, yes, but I support the people who love them just as much. Fear goes down. Clarity goes up. And suddenly everyone feels like they can handle what's coming.

By the time I leave that first visit, the ones who were most skeptical are often the first to hug me. They go from tight shoulders and held breath to soft eyes and relief. It's not because I convinced them of anything. It's because I saw them. And I saw the person at the center of all this long before I saw the diagnosis.

The real work is seeing the person, not just the process.

Doctors watch labs and scans.
Hospice balances comfort, visits, and a full roster of families who need them.
Loved ones grieve while the person is still alive.

My role is to sit in the middle of all of that and remember this is still a human being with preferences, personality, and agency. They are more than the dying process.

One of the first questions I ask is the simplest and also the most radical: "What do *you* want?"

That question changes everything. It hands power back to the person who has been slowly losing pieces of themselves to appointments, scans, procedures, hopes, and fears.

I've worked with clients who have done chemo for years, and no one ever asked them if they wanted to. Not once. They just kept saying yes to whatever came next, because that's what the system expects of people. More treatment. More fighting. More time.

But sometimes the person is exhausted. Sometimes they don't want to spend their last chapter fighting for more chapters at all. Asking, "What do you want?" can be the first time someone has a choice in months.

And then there are the tiny details. That's how you really learn who someone is.

I once had a client who wanted her hair to be the right color for her funeral. She colored it herself with henna for years, and a few weeks before she died, we sat together and did her hair. The house smelled like herbs and tea. She was weak, but she was smiling. She kept saying, "You know I have to look good, Kacie. Don't let me go out looking crazy with old lady hair."

That hair wasn't vanity. It was identity. It was dignity. It was her saying, "This is who I am. Let me be myself until the end."

Another client barely ate anything at all, but every single day she wanted her Starbucks iced coffee. Two teaspoons of sugar, half-and-half mixed in, ice clinking in the tumbler. She swore no one made it as good as I did, which is hilarious because I didn't do anything special. Her adult kids would call me saying, "Can you come make Mom a coffee? She says I don't do it right."

It wasn't about the coffee.
It was about ritual.
It was about pleasure.
It was about one tiny thing that made her feel alive.

Those little human details are the map to who someone is. Sometimes what reveals a person isn't what they want but what they refuse.

I once had a client who hadn't showered in two years. She had a stroke. She lived in a long-term care environment with staff and family rotating through to help. She could walk, she could get around, but the shower terrified her. Every attempt ended the same way: tears, shaking, clinging to the doorway like she was fighting for her life.

People had been trying to get her to shower for years. Staff tried. Family tried. Nobody knew why she was so afraid, and because she had aphasia, she couldn't explain it. Everyone assumed it was stubbornness.

No one realized it was fear.

But then one day she and I were watching a movie together, and there was a scene of someone drowning. She looked at me with tears in her eyes, pointed at the person drowning, and then pointed at her tracheostomy. The fear was all over her face.

That's when it hit me; she was terrified the shower would drown her.

No one had considered this. For two years, everyone offered showers, because that's what the facility had. No one offered a bath. They hadn't connected the dots. But in that one moment of shared understanding, everything changed. I asked gently, "Are you afraid you will drown in the shower?" She nodded "yes" furiously.

"Would you feel safe taking a bath instead?" Her whole body lit up. No hesitation. She nodded so fast I thought she might fall out of her chair.

I went to the facility and asked if there were any bathtubs she could use. Thankfully there was a whirlpool tub on a different floor, and they agreed to let her use it. I filled the tub with warm water, bubbles, safety. She sank into that bath like she had been waiting her whole life for it. She splashed. She washed her hair. She relaxed in a way I had never seen. And from that day on, she took baths regularly.

She didn't need motivation.
She needed someone to see her fear.
That's the work.
Seeing the person, not the resistance.

Seeing the human, not the diagnosis.
That's where everything shifts.

Sometimes the person gets lost inside the decline. Not because the family doesn't care, but because watching someone fade is unbearable. They start talking about the person like they're not in the room.

I once sat at a bedside where a husband answered every question for his wife. He was loving, but anxious. Protective, but suffocating. Every time I asked her something, he would jump in with, "She can't answer. She's out of breath. She gets tired."

I could see the frustration on her face. She was still here. She still had things to say. So, I smiled at him and said, "I love hearing your perspective. But I would love to hear her answer too. I have plenty of time. Even one-word answers are okay."

That small sentence changed the whole room. He backed up. He took a breath. And she got to speak for herself. She was relieved. Her shoulders dropped. She answered in short sentences, slowly, but with so much dignity. She was still her, and someone finally gave her space to be.

It's easy to lose the person in decline. But they are still there. Sometimes fully themselves, right up to the very end.

I've had clients crack jokes hours before they died. Clients who cussed like sailors. Clients who demanded a certain blanket, a certain pillow arrangement, a certain playlist, even when they could barely whisper.

I once sat with a woman whose room smelled like herbal tea and Vicks. Her favorite music was playing softly in the background, mixed with the rhythmic hissing of her oxygen concentrator. She was curled under the softest blanket in the world, covered in cute little kitty cats. The lights were off, sunlight spilling over the bed. That room was full of love and comfort and presence. It felt like her.

That's what surprises families the most:
They expect the dying to be gone.
But they are still here.

They still care about comfort, pleasure, agency, coffee, blankets, lipstick, hair dye, music, pets, who is sitting in the room, and who isn't. They still want to choose. They still want to laugh. They still want to be themselves.

Families often discover that their person is still living, even as they are dying. And that realization brings relief. It brings humanity back into the room.

Because at the center of every death is a person who matters, who has preferences, rituals, memories, pet peeves, humor, fear, and hope. They aren't done living just because they are dying.

Our job is to see that. And honor it.

When I teach my students how to meet clients for the first time, I tell them: "Don't go in asking, 'What's wrong?' Go in asking, 'What's top of mind for you today?'"

That is where trust begins.
That is where peace begins.
Every death is different.
Every person is different.

And every one of them deserves to be seen fully, not as a diagnosis or a decline but as a human being doing the most human thing any of us will ever do: leave this world.

The Family System

If you've ever walked into a house where someone is dying, you know immediately that you're stepping into more than one kind of grief. There's the grief for the person who's leaving, and then there's the grief for how everyone else is handling it or not handling it at all.

Every family becomes its own little ecosystem when death moves in. There's usually one person who refuses to accept what's happening, one person who's holding everything together with sheer willpower, and at least one person who copes by staying very, very busy. Sometimes, the one holding everything together is the very person who is dying.

Over time, you start to recognize the roles: the avoider, the doer, the fixer, the quiet one, the one who makes every decision, and the one who pretends there's no decision to make. The sibling who suddenly becomes an expert because they "Googled it." The brother who stands in the kitchen aggressively doing dishes so he doesn't have to cry. The daughter who keeps asking the same question in different ways because she's desperate for a different answer.

And almost always, the avoider hates me at first. Because bringing in a death doula is the moment it stops being hypothetical. It's no longer "someday, years from now." It's here. It's now. I am living, breathing confirmation that things are serious enough that they needed to call in someone with "death" in her job title.

The fear looks for somewhere to land. Sometimes it lands on me.

I've been glared at, ignored, complained about, and sized up more times than I can count. I've had people refuse to make eye contact with me for an entire visit. I've watched spouses fold their arms and sit as far away from me as the room allows. Early on, that used to rattle me. I'd go home wondering what I did wrong.

Now I know better. They're not mad at me. They're mad that life is not going the way they thought it would. They're mad that someone they love is dying and they can't fix it. I just happen to be the easiest target in the room.

I meet that resistance with patience and consistency. I don't push. I don't force trust. I show up on time. I keep my word. I care out loud. And nine times out of ten, the avoider is the one who ends up hugging me the hardest at the end.

One of the most beautiful family systems I've ever worked with was a woman who had been an RN herself. She was dying from cancer, but you would've thought she'd spent her entire career teaching people how to die well. She'd prepared her family with so much intention. They knew what medications she did and didn't want. They knew what kind of room she wanted to die in. Everyone knew her wishes, and no one was stuck in denial.

Her husband was her primary caregiver. Her three adult children rotated in and out of the hospice room, not as frantic caretakers but as a circle of love. They sat at her bedside telling old stories, laughing about childhood mishaps, crying when they needed to and not apologizing for it. They held her hand, brushed her hair, adjusted her blankets the way she liked them.

There was a harmony in that room that you can't fake.

It was in the way they spoke gently to one another. In the way someone always had a hand on her arm. In the way they talked to her like she was still there, not like she was already gone.

I remember commending them repeatedly on how beautiful it was. I even took photos of them together as she labored out of life (with their permission, of course). To an outsider, that might sound grim, but it wasn't. It was holy. I am convinced she was floating above us, watching with joy as her family did exactly what she'd hoped they would do: love each other well while they said goodbye to her.

She died peacefully, no panic, no fighting, no last-minute drama. Just presence.

That's what it looks like when a family understands what death really is: not just a loss to be feared but a transition to be honored.

But I've seen the other side, too.

I once worked with a woman in her early fifties who had lived through a lifetime of chaos. Her ex-husband had been abusive. Her children were estranged from one another. There was tension in every corner of that home, the kind you can feel in your jaw before anyone starts talking.

She told me early on, "All I want is to die in peace."

That became our shared goal.

However, peace wasn't something her family knew how to do. Chaos was their native language. During her final hours, her children started arguing. Not soft disagreements, full-volume, old-history, "you always do this!" kind of fighting. The ex-husband showed up and poured gasoline on the fire. Voices rose. Bodies tensed. The air in the room went from tender to explosive in minutes.

I could see her struggling to rest in the middle of it. Her breath got shallow. Her brow tightened. Her whole body looked like it was bracing for impact.

So, I did what any good doula would do: I cleared the room.

Calmly. Firmly. Without apology.

I asked three grown men to step out so she could have what she had asked for from the beginning: peace.

As the door closed behind them, the noise left with them. The room exhaled. I watched her shoulders and jaw soften, her breathing deepen. I leaned in and whispered, "I've got you. Remember? We said peaceful. I meant it." I swear I saw the faintest little smile at the edge of her lips.

That's the power families don't always realize they have. They shape the atmosphere of the deathbed more than any medication ever could.

I wish more people understood that hearing is the last sense to go. Even when someone seems deeply asleep or unresponsive, they can still hear you. They can feel the energy in the room. They can tell the difference between a fight and a story, between tension and tenderness.

So be intentional with what you bring into that space.

Arguing in the doorway? They hear that.
Whisper-fighting over the bed? They feel that.
Rehashing old wounds at the foot of the bed? They carry that.
On the other hand:

Telling them your favorite memory.
Thanking them for the way they loved you.
Reading their favorite book out loud.
Playing the song they used to dance to in the kitchen.
That lands, too.

I've watched pain ease just from the sound of laughter. I've watched a clenched jaw soften when a daughter starts singing to her mother. I've watched restless bodies relax when someone finally says the words they've been choking on for days: "It's okay to go. We're going to be okay."

I tell my students at Death Doula School: we have the ability to transform not just how people die but how families remember death itself. When a family can look back and say, "Yes, it was sad, but it was also beautiful," that's healing. That's legacy.

The hardest part of this job isn't the death itself; it's staying grounded in the middle of someone else's long, complicated story. You will sit with families who are still playing out dynamics that started decades ago. You'll watch people try to argue about things that happened in 1994 while their loved one is taking their last breaths.

You can't fix that. You're not there to be the family therapist, the referee, or the judge. You're there to protect the person at the center and the integrity of the space around them as best you can.

Sometimes that means gently redirecting:

> "Let's bring it back to her. What would feel comforting to her right now?"

Sometimes it means naming what you're seeing:

> "I can tell everyone here is really scared. What would be most helpful in this moment, for her?"

Sometimes it means saying less and breathing more, letting your calm body be the thing that lowers the volume in the room.

Families will project their fear, their guilt, their love, their denial, all of it, onto the deathbed. Our job isn't to judge it. It's to hold steady so they have something solid to lean on while everything else feels like it's falling apart.

Because no matter how chaotic it gets, the truth remains:
Death reveals people. It brings out the best, the worst, and everything in between.

And when you can meet all of it with compassion and neutrality, you help turn even the most tangled family system into something that, in its own imperfect way, is still sacred.

In the next section, we'll zoom in even closer, not just on who the family members are but on the emotional landscapes they bring with them. Fear, anger, guilt, relief, love, denial, it all shows up at the bedside. Understanding those emotions is just as important as understanding the people who carry them.

The Emotional Landscapes They Bring

When I walk into a new case, the air in the room almost always feels the same at first. It's thick. Heavy. The emotional temperature is visible before anyone speaks. There's grief for the person who is dying, and then there's grief for how everyone else is handling it. . .or not handling it at all. People don't know where to look. They don't know what to do with their hands. They're terrified of doing it wrong. And how could they know? There isn't exactly a manual for this. (Well. . .until now.)

I walk in the door with calm because my nervous system sets the tone. If I show up flustered, they'll meet me there. If I show up grounded, they'll eventually settle. You can feel it happen in real time; someone takes a deep breath they didn't realize they were holding. Sometimes the whole room does, like the moment you open a window in a stuffy house.

The emotional landscape of death is never one thing. It's a kaleidoscope, constantly shifting. Fear sits right next to love. Sadness and gratitude trade places. Someone is laughing in the kitchen while someone else is crying in the hallway. And underneath it all is this quiet hum of disbelief that a life is ending in this house.

People expect death to feel only tragic. But it doesn't. Maybe convert to feelings. . .it feels. . .there is laughter. There are jokes. There is relief. There is guilt. There is peace.

One of the most heartbreaking and beautiful emotional patterns I ever witnessed came from a woman with brain cancer. She had been planning her death for almost two years, ever since the day she got that terrifying diagnosis: glioblastoma. She was precise, meticulous, organized in a way that made my doula heart sing. She wanted everything to be intentional. She wanted her family prepared.

She hired me early, before hospice, before decline, because she wanted someone who would help her think through every step. Together, we held meetings with her sisters, her kids, her closest friends. We sat at her dining room table with calendars and cups of tea and talked about what she wanted and what she didn't. We interviewed hospice teams and chose the one that aligned with her values. She wasn't just ready; she was leading the way.

Her husband loved her very much, but he also refused to participate. He was devastated. Furious. Not at her but at cancer, at fate, at the doctors, at a universe that had the audacity to take the woman he loved. Avoidance became his coping strategy. He would walk into the room, see us planning, and walk right back out. He didn't want to hear anything that sounded like goodbye.

When she began to decline, cognition slipped the way it often does with brain cancer. She could no longer make every decision herself. And suddenly, the husband who had refused to be involved became the one holding the power. Hospice was brought up by her doctors once the treatments were no longer working. He refused. My involvement was brought up. He refused. He refused everything that acknowledged reality. He wasn't ready to let her go, so he denied her plan that he resented so much.

When I got the call that she died, I was sitting in my car. I cried. Not because she died; we had expected that. I cried because she had planned so beautifully, and then it was taken from her at the end. Love can look like control when we are drowning.

That's the emotional landscape of death. Love, fear, control, avoidance, tenderness all mixed into one.

Another emotional landscape shows up at the moment of death. People don't realize how long the active dying phase can last. The body can take days to shut down. Sometimes more than a week. Families sit vigil, watching breath by breath, waiting. It is exhausting. It is sacred. It is brutal.

I have seen people cry and exhale at the exact same moment. A son once said, with tears streaming down his face, "I'm so sad. . .and I'm so relieved at the same time." He felt guilty for the relief, but relief is human. Watching someone slowly slip away is a marathon. The finish line brings grief and mercy.

And then there are the flashes of absurd, hilarious humanity that sneak in through the cracks. I once worked with a woman and her adult daughter. We were cleaning out boxes, deciding what to donate. We were being serious and responsible. Then we opened a box of unopened face masks. She lit up.

"Stop everything," she said. "We are doing these right now. I am not going to my grave looking haggard."

So that's what we did. We stopped sorting, sat around her bed, put on face masks, and laughed with our ridiculous spa-day faces. One week later, she died. Her daughter told me, "I'll never look at a face mask again without smiling."

That's death. It's tender. It's funny. It's holy. It's human.

Children in the house bring their own emotional weather. They see things adults try to avoid. I've had little girls look straight at a dying grandparent and ask, "Are you dying?" No fear. Just curiosity. I swear, some of them are tiny doulas in training.

One woman I worked with had an 11-year-old daughter. As she declined, she grew too weak to get out of bed. So, they made the bed their world. The daughter painted her nails, did her makeup, brushed her hair. When she died, that little girl climbed into bed and painted her mother's nails one last time so she could "go to heaven with a fresh mani-pedi." Kids understand more than we give them credit for.

Not every landscape is peaceful. Sometimes peace is blocked by fear. I sat with a woman who was deeply holistic and wellness-minded. She wanted hospice medication, but her husband refused because he believed it would "make her die faster." She suffered for weeks, restless, anxious, unable to rest.

One afternoon, she looked at me and whispered, "I want the medicine. He won't let me."

So, I sat with them and explained, calmly, clearly, compassionately, that the medication wasn't going to cause her death. It was going to release her from suffering. She turned to her husband and said, "Please. I need this." He finally agreed. That evening, she got her first dose. Her body relaxed. Her breath slowed. Her face softened. For the first time in weeks, she looked peaceful.

Sometimes peace is not about changing death. It's about changing fear.

Being a doula means you walk into the storm and become the calm. You don't stop the weather. You steady it. You hold the container so everyone else can crumble safely.

But you don't carry it home. You can witness their grief without swallowing it. Before I enter a home, I pause at the door. I take a deep breath. I leave my own life outside. When I leave, I hand back whatever belongs to them. If I don't, I end up carrying the echo of every room I've ever sat in. That echo becomes tension in my jaw, snapping at my kids, staring at my phone, and not seeing anything.

Empathy makes us good at this work. Boundaries keep us in it.

The emotional landscapes families bring are not something to fix. They are something to honor. Every emotion, anger, relief, joy, fear is part of the story. When a doula stays steady, the family finds steadiness too.

And that steadiness is what shapes memory. When a family can look back and say, "It was sad and hard. . .and it was beautiful," that is healing. That is legacy. We don't just support the dying. We support the living in how they will remember the dying.

None of these emotional landscapes is a problem. They are the truth of being human. And when we can meet all of it, the rage, the laughter, the relief, the tenderness with compassion and neutrality, we turn chaos into something sacred.

That is the emotional work. And from here, we can go deeper.

Because emotions don't arrive alone. They come from history, relationships, culture, identity.

That means death doesn't just happen to one person; it happens to the whole ecosystem.

And that's where we go next.

The Doula's Role Within These Systems

The role of a death doula inside a family system is quieter than people think. There's no entrance music. No "ta-da." If you do it well, no one can quite explain what you did, only that something felt different when you were there. The air felt calmer. People breathed deeper. The room stopped feeling like it might explode.

When I walk into a home, I am not just walking into a house where someone is dying. I am walking into a whole ecosystem. A history. A decade's worth of unresolved conflicts. Old resentments. Inside jokes. Family roles that have been carved in stone since childhood.

Most families have their cast of characters.
The avoider. The fixer. The planner. The jokester. I am not there to rearrange the cast. I am there to sit in the middle of them and keep the stage from collapsing.

One of the clearest examples of this was a mother I worked with who was estranged from one of her adult sons. She was dying and she wanted him there. That was the one thing she kept circling back to.

Not her bucket list, not a grand trip, not some dramatic final gesture. She just wanted her boy in the room.

They had butted heads for years. I'm sure the backstory was complicated. What I knew was this: he had pulled away for his own reasons, and being her son did not erase those reasons.

She asked me to reach out to him. I told her I would, but I also told her I would not pressure him. Whatever he chose, I would respect it and support him through it. She agreed.

He was only 18. That is such a young age to be asked to walk into a deathbed and reconcile a lifetime. When I spoke with him, he was kind but firm. He told me he had no intention of coming, not now and not later. He understood she was dying. He understood people thought he might regret it. He still said no.

And then there was the other brother, furious that his sibling would not show up. He wanted me to convince him. To shame him. To "make him see sense."

I could not do that either. I held three truths at the same time:
A dying mother grieving the son who would not come.
A son protecting himself from something the rest of us could not understand.
Another son enraged on everyone's behalf.

I did not fix it. I did not reunite them. I did not manufacture a Hallmark ending.

I listened. I validated each of their perspectives. I reminded the 18-year-old that he was still worthy of support and care even if he could not show up the way others wanted him to. I reminded the brother that his anger made sense and would not change his sibling's choice. I reminded the mother that her son's absence did not erase his love, or hers. One of the doula's roles inside a system is neutrality. Not coldness. Not distance. Neutrality as love that stretches wide enough to hold everyone without collapsing in the middle.

Sometimes being neutral means standing in the emotional hallway and refusing to be dragged into one room or the other. Families will try to recruit you. They will say things like, “Tell him he’s wrong,” or “You see what I mean, right?” And honestly, sometimes I do see it. Sometimes I agree completely. But that is not my job.

My job is not to take sides. My job is to keep the hallway open so they can still walk toward each other if they ever decide to. Other times, my role is to be the only calm nervous system present.

I have walked into homes where everyone was in full meltdown. People pacing. Someone sobbing in the bathroom. Someone else barking orders. The dying person in the bed, absorbing all of it, too tired to say, “Please stop.”

In those rooms, my first tool is always my own body. Slow breath. Soft shoulders. Steady voice. No rush.

You can almost feel the room lean toward that. Our nervous systems are contagious. If I come in frantic, they will spike higher. If I come in grounded, they eventually start to match me.

Sometimes that looks very practical.
“Let’s all sit for a second.”
“Take a sip of water.”
“Let’s slow this down and make sure we’re keeping her comfortable.”

One simple line, said with confidence, can drop the emotional temperature 10 degrees. Other times, the most meaningful thing I do looks like nothing at all from the outside.

I think often of a woman with lung cancer who was terrified of the actual moment of death, but not afraid to talk about it. Her family could not tolerate those conversations. Any time she named her reality, they shut it down.

“Don’t say that.”
“Stay positive.”
“We’re still hoping for a miracle.”

She did not want a miracle. She wanted honesty. She wanted companionship at the edge.

She told me, “I only feel like I can be myself when you are here.”

As she declined, she asked for my presence more and more. Talking became harder. She hated being questioned or pushed to speak. So many visitors meant well, but they exhausted her. They came in like cheerleaders when what she needed was a witness. So, I became the witness.

In the final weeks, our visits were mostly quiet. She lay in bed, breath shallow, eyes half-closed. I sat beside her. I held her hand. I stroked her hair. Sometimes I hummed. Sometimes I did nothing at all.

Every so often, she would squeeze my hand and whisper, "Don't leave yet." So I stayed.

If you had walked by the door, you might have thought nothing was happening. No dramatic conversation. No big spiritual revelation. Just a woman in a bed and another woman in a chair.

Inside that silence, everything was happening.
She was dying the way she needed to die.
Seen. Not gaslit. Not told to "fight." Just held.

That is the doula's role too: to hold space.

And then there are moments when the room desperately needs someone to name what is happening and make a clear call.

I remember a man whose wife had always hated his cat. Truly hated it. This cat had arrived by way of the "cat distribution system" and she never forgave it. The feeling was mutual. The cat kept its distance.

On her last day, she was hours from death. The house was quiet. Everyone was tired. And out of nowhere, this cat hopped up onto the bed, as if someone had called it in. It walked along the edge of her body, sniffing, taking her in. Then it curled up against her side and went to sleep.

Her husband and I just stared.

We both knew, if she had been awake and herself, she would have lost her mind about that cat touching her blankets. We whispered back and forth about how mad she would be if she knew. We laughed in that hushed, disbelieving way you laugh in church when you know you shouldn't.

I was about to move the cat, but I wanted to see what it would do. It sniffed her hand, then licked it, then settled back down. She moved one finger, the tiniest motion, as if she were petting it.

So, we left the cat there.

The woman who hated that animal spent her last hours with it curled against her side, the two of them keeping each other warm. There was humor in that. There was tenderness too. There was a kind of quiet mystery I still cannot fully explain.

That is another part of the doula's role inside these systems: letting the weird, holy, unplanned moments happen. Not over-managing. Not making everything precious and serious. Letting the cat stay on the bed.

At the heart of this job is support.
Not just support for the sweet, tidy, well-behaved parts of people, but support for all of it.

Support for the husband who is angry at death and needs somewhere to put that anger.
Support for the daughter painting her mom's nails in bed because that is how she can still feel useful.
Support for the son who cannot come back and the brother who cannot understand why.
Support for the dying person who just wants someone to sit down, shut up, and hold their hand.

The doula's role is not to fix families.
The doula's role is to hold them as they are and create enough steadiness that something softens.

We do not control outcomes. We influence the atmosphere.

We are not the main character in the story.
We are the grounded presence who helps everyone else survive the chapter.

When I think about what it really means to work inside these systems, it comes down to this: support in the loud moments and the quiet ones, through the fights and the reconciliations and the silences that never get resolved. To be a calm body in the room—a clear voice when people need guidance and a witness when there is nothing left to say.

And once we understand this, once we know how to hold space for the person, the family, and the emotional weather they bring, the next question becomes: how do we pull it all together in practice, from the first conversation to the final goodbye?

That is where we go next.

Bringing It All Together

When I step back and look at the people I've served, the dying, their families, the circles of chaos and love that form around them, one thing becomes clearer every year: death doulas are the steady thread that holds it all together. We are the anchor when the world begins to tilt. We are the ones who walk into the storm without trying to stop the weather, only to guide everyone through it.

We're the steady presence in the middle of uncertainty. The calm voice when fear takes over. We can sit at a bedside at 3 a.m. when everyone else has gone home because they couldn't bear to watch anymore. We stand in the doorway between what is and what's coming next, not as gatekeepers but as companions. And because of that, we have the power to change the way the world experiences death. Not someday. Now.

Most people assume our job begins when the dying person is already unresponsive. They think we're brought in to hold a hand at the final breath, whisper a few sweet words, and drive off into the moonlight like a Hallmark character in black scrubs. But that is the tiniest sliver of what we do. The real work happens long before the last breath. The real work happens in kitchens and living rooms, on couches and back porches, in quiet conversations and shared silence. We show up months before the end, sometimes longer. We help people live while they're still living.

We don't stop the dying. We stop the panic around death.

When I was a nurse, death felt like failure. It was what happened when nothing else worked. But becoming a death doula changed everything. Death isn't failure. It's transition. It's sacred. It's human. When families are supported, when the person who is dying is allowed to live right up to the final moment, something profound happens: fear steps aside, and love moves in. The room changes. The air changes. You can feel it.

I've stood in rooms where people held hands and told stories for hours. I've been in rooms where laughter erupted at the bedside because someone made a joke in their last hours and everyone needed that release so badly. I've held space for daughters painting their mother's nails, for husbands brushing hair, for dogs curled up against a chest they loved. I have seen the most ordinary moments become holy. This is not the part of death people imagine, but it's real. It's tender. It's beautiful.

People think they are preparing for a death, but what they are really preparing for is a memory.

Death is not just the end of a person; it is the beginning of a story that will live in the minds of everyone who loved them.

If every dying person had a death doula, every family would have support, every ending would be held with love instead of confusion, we would live in a culture that doesn't fear death so much. Imagine a world where children grow up watching death handled with tenderness. Imagine a generation that doesn't hide from grief but learns how to companion it. Imagine adults who don't view hospice as "giving up," but as permission to focus on comfort, on connection, on meaning.

We could change everything. Not in theory, in practice. We already are.

When I step into a home where someone is dying, I always bring one thing with me more than anything else: presence. Not solutions. Not answers. Not a fix. Just presence. Sometimes that is all that's needed. A hand on a shoulder. A warm blanket. A quiet voice that says, "You're safe. We're here."

I tell people all the time that my job isn't to pull anyone out of grief. My job is to sit with them inside it so they don't feel alone. I watch families take their first deep breath in days because someone finally acknowledged what is happening. I see peace settle into rooms that were tight with anxiety. I see bodies relax, tears fall, shoulders soften. I see the moment when control is finally surrendered, and trust appears.

This work teaches us that we don't just help people die. We help them live all the way through it. We help them design their final chapter. We give them autonomy in a world that often strips it away. We protect the space so that the people who love them can grieve and laugh and say goodbye without being swallowed whole by fear.

Every time I leave a home after someone has died, I stand outside for a moment. I breathe. I look at the trees, or the sky, or the quiet street. Life continues. There is always a bird singing or a car passing or snow falling gently on the windshield. And I remember: this is the point. Death is not separate from life. It is woven into it.

And that is why I do this. Not to witness death. But to witness life.

CHAPTER 5

The Roles of the Doula

People always ask me, "So. . .what exactly does a death doula do?"

I've tried giving short answers. I've tried giving long answers. I've tried metaphors, diagrams, jokes, and once even mimed the shape of a roller coaster, which honestly was probably the most accurate portrayal I've ever offered. But the truth is this:

> **We do the same thing birthing doulas do, just on the other end of life.**

We help someone plan, prepare, and move through one of the most sacred transitions a human will ever experience. We help them shape their final chapter, honor their values, and meet death on their own terms.

But the *real* answer? It depends on the day. Sometimes, it depends on the minute.

Some days, I am a teacher, explaining the dying process the way another person might explain how to assemble IKEA furniture, calmly, step-by-step, without using the word "doom" even once. Other days, I'm a grief counselor, a spiritual companion, a logistics coordinator, a fierce advocate, a translator between hospice and family, or the referee in the middle of a generational trauma cage match.

Some days I'm the strong one.
Some days I'm the soft one.
Some days I'm both before breakfast.

Nothing about this job fits neatly into a box, which is exactly what makes it so powerful.

Every doula brings their own background and magic to the table. I came from nursing. I've stood at thousands of bedsides in scrubs, charting vitals, managing symptoms, and watching systems fail while families tried their best to understand what was happening. Now I walk in without the stethoscope, but with something different, the human side of care, the part that never fit into the medical framework in the first place.

Other doulas come from social work, massage therapy, chaplaincy, energy work, Reiki, therapy, teaching, salon work, or no professional background at all. I once trained a doula who had been a software engineer for 32 years. She left tech because one of her parents died without support, and she couldn't stand the idea of anyone else going through that alone. Two years later, she built a digital legacy tool that helped her clients record their life stories. People carry gifts into this calling that they don't even know are gifts yet.

There is no one right path into this work.
The common thread is heart.
And within that heart, doulas wear many hats, often all at once.

I'll never forget the night I got a call from two young women in their early twenties. Their mom was in the hospital with terminal cancer, and the nurse on duty refused to give her the pain medication that was ordered. They called her a "drug seeker." A dying woman. Diagnosed with a terminal cancer diagnosis. Labeled that way.

They were sobbing when they called me. They didn't know what to do. They were watching their mother suffer and had no power to stop it. Within thirty minutes, I was in my car, driving through the dark, adrenaline and instinct doing all the work.

When I walked into that hospital room, I wasn't just the doula anymore. I was the educator, explaining terminal pain and comfort care.

I was the advocate, firm but calm, insisting the nurse follow the physician's orders or call someone who would.
I was emotional support for two daughters who had been holding their breath for hours.
And when the medication was finally given and the pain eased, I was the witness, standing in the soft quiet as their mother's body unfurled like a fist finally opening.

We wear many hats. Sometimes, we wear all of them within a single hour.

New doulas always imagine the job like this: you sit at the bedside for days on end, holding someone's hand until their final breath. They ask me, "But how do you do that with kids?" or "Do you just stay there the whole time?" That's the version people picture because that's the part movies show.

But real death work is more dynamic than that.

The active dying phase can last three to fourteen days, sometimes more. You cannot physically sit at a bedside nonstop for that long, and more importantly, that's not what families need or expect. You visit, you guide, you support, you offer presence when it's needed and space when it's appropriate. You adjust your rhythm to theirs. Some days you're there for an hour. Some days you return twice. Some days what they need most is a phone call at midnight to confirm that the breathing pattern they're seeing is normal.

It's not about clocking hours.
It's about meeting the moment.
And every moment is different.

Flexibility is survival in this work; emotional flexibility especially. You have to be able to move from heartbreak to humor to logistics to advocacy without losing your footing. I've gone from comforting a spouse who believes their partner can still recover. . .to stepping into the kitchen to help another family member understand what an oxygen drop means. . .to cracking a gentle joke five minutes later to keep someone from falling apart.

Some people think humor doesn't belong at the end of life. I disagree completely. Humor brings breath back into a tight room. Humor reopens the nervous system. Humor reminds people they are still alive and still connected. If you've followed my social media for even five minutes, you know I'll joke all the way to the grave. Literally.

The truth is, not everyone is built for this kind of work. It takes a strange blend of softness and steel. You have to feel things deeply without collapsing under them. You have to walk into a room vibrating with fear and somehow lower the frequency to something the human body can survive. You have to be comfortable in silence. You have to be unbothered by tears. You have to be willing to say "death" out loud in a world that whispers it like a curse word.

That's what sets death doulas apart from nurses, chaplains, social workers, therapists, and well-meaning family members. We bring something different, a quiet, grounded presence paired with deep emotional intelligence. We don't come in with a protocol. We come in with intuition. We can shift the energy in a room without anyone noticing what we did. We can catch a fear before it becomes panic. We can anchor a family with nothing more than steady breath and a soft tone.

We are not built like everyone else.
We are built for this.
And whether we call it a calling, a knowing, or simply who we've always been, the truth is the same:

> **We were made to walk with people through the end, and whatever comes after.**

Advocacy: The Voice for the Voiceless

Advocacy is one of the most misunderstood parts of death doula work. People hear the word and immediately picture someone charging down a hospital hallway, voice raised, ready to fight. And sure, sometimes advocacy does look like that. Sometimes you do have to walk into a room with your shoulders squared and your voice steady and say, "This isn't acceptable." But most of the time, advocacy is quieter. It's strategic. It's relational. It's one human being standing between another human being and the suffering they shouldn't have to endure.

Being an advocate comes in a lot of shapes and colors. Sometimes I'm standing up to a healthcare system that's failing my client. Other times I'm helping someone find their voice inside their own family. Sometimes I am the only person in the room willing to name the thing everyone else is too scared to say out loud. And often, I'm teaching people how to advocate for themselves. How to stop doing what everyone else wants and start asking for what they want. That's the heart of advocacy in this work: giving power back to the dying person in a world that has been stripping it away one appointment, one form, one prognosis at a time.

And the truth is, I didn't learn how to advocate as a doula. I learned it as a nurse, long before I knew this work existed, long before I understood how much the skill of speaking up would matter. My foundation for advocacy was built in those fluorescent hallways, at hospital bedsides, in moments when I knew someone needed a voice and no one else was stepping up. One story still lives in my bones, because it taught me the difference one determined person can make.

I had a patient with cancer, a sweet man with a developmental delay who trusted anyone in scrubs like they were family. Once chemo started, he stopped eating. Completely. Nothing worked. Not coaxing. Not bargaining. Not positive reinforcements or rewards. Not even a milkshake from McDonald's, which had been his holy grail of joy.

I knew he wasn't refusing food to be defiant. He was sick. Miserable. Lost in a body that suddenly betrayed him. Around that same time, I had just learned about a medication called Marinol, a synthetic THC that early research showed could help stimulate appetite. FDA-approved. Safe. Absolutely worth trying.

Now keep in mind, this was *many years ago*, back when anything related to marijuana still made doctors flinch. We were just beginning to understand the medical benefits, and there was still a whole lot of stigma attached to it. Suggesting Marinol back then did *not* land the way it lands today.

I brought it to the doctor, hopeful. He brushed me off.

"I'm not going to be the doctor who prescribes marijuana," he said, with a smirk that made it clear the conversation was over. But I wasn't done.

I went home that night and did what every good advocate does: I built a case. I pulled research, studies, clinical data. I printed everything I could find and highlighted the hell out of it. I marched back to him with a stack of papers and the conviction of someone who knew exactly what her patient needed. He finally relented.

Two days after starting the medication, my patient walked to the nurses' station for the first time in weeks asking for breakfast. Then lunch. Then dinner. Then a milkshake.

He smiled again. He joked again. He was *alive* again.

That moment taught me something I've carried into every corner of my doula work: **advocacy is not about volume; it's about persistence. It's about refusing to look away when someone is suffering.**

But advocacy doesn't always end in victory. Some stories stay with you because you fought and won. Others haunt you because you fought and lost.

I once cared for a woman with dementia, the kind of dementia that makes the world feel like a foreign country. She had days where she was combative, terrified, confused, trapped in a body that could no longer translate what she felt. Staff labeled these moments as "behaviors." I labeled them as suffering.

I had this feeling she needed hospice. I could feel it in my bones. She was declining rapidly, losing weight, withdrawing, fluctuating between agitation and collapse. But hospice eligibility for dementia requires a very specific set of criteria, and she didn't check the right boxes. Her doctor kept saying, "She's not near the end." I kept saying, "Yes, she is."

I begged for a hospice consult. I documented everything. I asked again. And again. And again.

Denied. Every time. Then one day, she went quiet.

No fighting, no resisting, no pushing away care. Just silence. That eerie calm that tells you the body has finally surrendered. She died three days later. Hospice arrived 24 hours before her death, far too late to provide the comfort and dignity she deserved.

That one still hurts.

Advocating and losing is a gut punch. But it also reshapes you. It teaches you what not to forget. It makes you fiercer, clearer, steadier. It's why today, as a doula, when a client says, "Something doesn't feel right," I listen like my life depends on it. Because theirs does.

Some advocacy moments are loud. Others are quiet, so quiet you'd miss them if you weren't paying attention.

I once worked with a woman in her forties with MS. She was bed-bound, unable to shower alone, vulnerable in every possible way. Her husband visited often, bringing their daughter with him. Staff whispered that he wasn't "nice," but whispers don't prepare you for the truth.

One day he visited her alone, without their daughter. I noticed her door was closed, unusual for her. My gut pinged. I knocked, walked in under the guise of doing nurse things, and found her husband assaulting her. She was frozen, crying silently.

I didn't yell. I didn't storm. I didn't lose control. Advocacy in that moment wasn't a roar; it was a laser-sharp, protective instinct.

"Out," I said. "Now."

Security removed him from the building.

I sat beside her afterward and gently asked if she had wanted him there. She said no. Asked if she was afraid of him. She said yes. Asked if she still wanted visits from him. She said no, but he was the only way she got to see her daughter.

So, I called social work. We found another family member willing to bring her daughter weekly. She was protected. She was safe. She had a choice again. Her husband was banned from visiting her anymore, but she still got to see her daughter regularly.

People imagine advocacy as "fighting the system," but sometimes it's this: **protecting someone whose voice has been silenced by fear, illness, or power imbalance.**

And then there's the advocacy that isn't loud or dramatic at all, the advocacy that looks like teaching.

I once worked with a woman in her early sixties who needed hospice, but her insurance didn't cover end-of-life services. At all. The cost? Over $900 a day. She wasn't old enough for Medicare. She didn't have Medicaid. And she didn't have the money to pay privately.

She had stage-four lung cancer and couldn't breathe, couldn't move, couldn't speak full sentences without being short of breath. We tried going through her primary doctor for home oxygen. They refused without an oxygen test. She went to the hospital. The test didn't dip low enough. They denied her again.

She sobbed in frustration. "I just want to breathe."

We tried something different.

We advocated quietly, together. She asked her doctor again. He blew her off. Finally, I asked her permission to step in. She handed me the phone like she was handing over her last piece of hope.

Twelve hours later, she had oxygen delivered to her home.

That wasn't loud advocacy. That was *strategic* advocacy, knowing when to nudge instead of push, when to soften instead of insist, when to speak in a doctor's language instead of your own.

And that is the art of advocacy: learning when to be the megaphone and when to be the microphone.

In doula work, I don't jump in at every moment. I don't take over. I don't speak for someone unless they ask. My rule is simple:

> **I don't intervene unless someone's safety, comfort, or autonomy is threatened or unless they explicitly ask me to be their voice.**

Otherwise, I support them in finding their own voice. Because advocacy that empowers someone to speak for themselves is one of the most beautiful parts of this work.

What I wish healthcare workers understood is that doulas aren't trying to disrupt the medical system. We're trying to *bridge* it. We fill the gaps they don't see. We hear the whispers they don't catch. We sit in the rooms they don't have time to sit in. We understand the fears patients won't say to their faces.

We're not here to replace anyone. We're here to make the whole thing work better, for everyone.

When advocacy is done right, it doesn't look like heroism. It looks like love in motion. It looks like someone finally breathing easier. It looks like a daughter saying, "Thank you. . .no one else fought for us." It looks like reduced suffering. Increased dignity. A final chapter written with intention instead of chaos.

True advocacy is not loudness. It's loyalty.

It is showing up again and again.
It is seeing the person no one else sees.
It is holding the line when systems fail.
It is the courage to speak and the wisdom to step back.
Advocacy, at its core, is this:

> **I won't let you go through this alone.**
>
> **Not your pain. Not your fear. Not your last chapter.**

The Four Pillars of Support

A good death doula holds up four corners of the same sacred space, **emotional, practical, spiritual, and logistical support.** These are what I call the *four pillars*. If even one is missing, things fall apart. When all four are working, the whole experience of death shifts for the dying person *and* their family.

EMOTIONAL SUPPORT

Emotional support isn't about "making someone feel better." It's about giving them permission to feel everything.

At the end of life, people start unpacking the whole closet of their lives: guilt, shame, regret, grief, relief, love, all of it. We want them to unpack it, because people die more peacefully when they're not carrying all that heaviness inside. But to do that, they have to feel completely safe with you. That's where holding space comes in.

Holding space means no judgment, no shocked face, no moral commentary. You just hold it all, with love.

I once had a client who was at the end of her life. We'd spent months together, and I could tell as death drew near that something was sitting heavy on her. I encouraged her to let it out so she could be more comfortable. She told me she hadn't spoken these words in more than 60 years. I held her hand and told her she was safe, that no matter what she told me, I wasn't going anywhere.

She told me that when she was a child, she was abused by her father in every way imaginable. At 18, her father forced her to marry one of his friends, who went on to abuse her the same way. She became pregnant, fell into postpartum depression, and when she tried to recover, her husband forced himself on her again. Two babies in two years, both born into violence.

One night, she packed what she could and ran. She disappeared, leaving her husband, and the babies, behind. She said it was either that or she would take her own life. Years later, when the children were adults, she tried to reconnect, but they wanted nothing to do with her.

She sobbed as she told me this, terrified that I would see her as a monster. But I didn't. I hugged her. I let her cry on my shoulder. That's holding space. Not fixing. Not judging. Just loving someone exactly as they are, so they can finally unburden themselves before they go.

That's emotional support. And it's sacred.

Sometimes it's not even about the big stories. Sometimes it's about silence. I once sat with a wife who'd been caregiving for months. Her husband was actively dying. People kept telling her, "You're so strong." She didn't need that. She just needed to not perform strength for once. I sat next to her, quiet. After a while, she whispered, "I don't want to do this part." And I said, "I know. You don't have to like it to do it well." That was it. She exhaled, and for the first time in days, she stopped clenching her jaw.

When things get really heavy in a room, I'll ground the energy with breathwork or guided imagery. I'll say, "Let's take a breath together," and lead them through a slow inhale and a longer exhale. Or I'll say, "Picture your feet on the floor. Picture roots growing down into the earth. You're safe. You can do this." Simple always works.

At Death Doula School, I teach that your face has to be safe, your voice has to be safe, and your silence has to be safe. That's emotional support in its truest form.

PRACTICAL SUPPORT

This is where the emotional meets the physical. Practical support is about turning a house into a sanctuary.

I help my clients create what I call their **hospice room**, the space where they'll spend their final days. We walk through the house together and choose the right room. Closest to the bathroom. No stairs. Enough space for a hospital bed. Once we've got the room, we make it *theirs*.

Sometimes we paint the walls a softer color. Sometimes we hang family photos. I am always careful to do things like remove rugs and clutter to prevent falls. Families always want to help, and this is where they can. I give them real jobs: clearing furniture, setting up the diffuser, washing blankets, creating a playlist of favorite songs. When people have something tangible to do, they feel calmer.

But practical support goes way beyond rearranging furniture. It's also about managing the life that's still happening around the dying process. I help my clients line up whatever additional help they might need, a dog walker, a house cleaner, someone to do the laundry or pick up groceries, a caregiver for respite hours. Sometimes I'm not just the doula, I'm the project manager of their end of life. I take the stress off their shoulders so they can focus on *living* while they're still here. Sometimes practical support looks like rearranging an entire house. And sometimes. . .it looks like grilled cheese.

I once worked with a client and his daughter, a daughter who had planned her dream vacation more than a year before her dad started to decline. She'd saved for it, counted down to it, dreamed about it. And now, months later, the timing collided with her father's worsening health. She was torn: go and feel guilty or stay and feel resentful. A classic end-of-life sandwich, where nobody wins and everybody feels terrible.

"But you'll be here, right?" she asked me one day, eyes wide like she was asking permission to breathe.

"Yes," I told her. "I'll check on him every day. And I'll keep you updated. You won't be abandoning him."

Still, she hesitated. Her dad was needy (her words, not mine), and she worried that as soon as she left, he would latch onto me the way he latched onto her. She pictured me spending hours by his bedside every visit, tending to every comfort, managing every little crisis.

But that man. . .oh, he was a character. And he didn't need emotional hand-holding or hour-long sit-downs. He needed lunch.

The first time I visited while she was away, he looked at me, pointed toward the kitchen, and said, "You make grilled cheese?"

I laughed. "Sir, grilled cheese is my love language."

The next day, it was sloppy joes. The day after that, back to grilled cheese. This man was consistent if nothing else.

Those small visits, those sandwiches, that normalcy, were exactly what he needed. Not a four-hour vigil. Not a deep emotional unraveling. Just someone who would show up, check in, and slap a slice of American cheese between two pieces of bread like it was the holiest ritual on Earth.

And for his daughter? Those simple visits were what allowed her to *go*. To take that trip. To step out of caregiver mode for a moment and remember she had a life too.

Practical support doesn't always look profound. But it *is* profound. Sometimes it's a freshly made bed. Sometimes it's picking up prescriptions or taking out the trash.

And sometimes, it's grilled cheese that keeps a whole family afloat.

New doulas often misunderstand this kind of work. They think the practical parts, rearranging rooms, organizing paperwork, calling the plumber, or coordinating caregivers, are somehow "less meaningful." They're not. These small, hands-on acts *are* the sacred work. You can't hold emotional space if everyone is overwhelmed because the laundry's piling up, the dog hasn't been walked, and no one has eaten dinner.

Practical support is what turns the dying process from crisis management into intentional care. It's not glamorous, but it's life-changing.

SPIRITUAL SUPPORT

I tell people all the time: death is spiritual, whether you're religious or not.

Even the most skeptical people start experiencing things at the end that they can't quite explain. Families sometimes panic when this happens. They'll whisper, "She's hallucinating," or "She keeps saying she sees her mom." And I'll calmly say, "That's normal. She's half here and half there. A little between this world, and whatever comes next."

I've seen this countless times. Almost all my clients see angels or loved ones before they die. They often describe them standing in doorways or closets. I had worked with one woman for almost eight months. She talked about her late husband constantly, Bob. She talked about Bob so much that I felt like I knew him too. As she neared death, I told her one day, "Don't be surprised if Bob shows up to get you and walk you home."

She opened her eyes wide and, with what little strength she had, whispered, "Bob is already here. He's been here for two days. He's sitting on the couch."

Of course, I looked at the couch hoping to see the ghost of Bob, I mean, you can't *not* look, but all I saw was an empty cushion. She smiled the softest smile and said the sentence I will never forget:

> "He says he's so happy to finally meet you in person."

I got chills that day. I have chills now, even telling it again. I couldn't see him, but I was honored to finally "meet" him too. I know he was there with her, in some way. You could feel the room shift, not spooky, not dramatic, just. . .softer. Like someone else had quietly walked in.

Moments like that remind me that death is not the end. It's a transition. A return. A crossing-over into something we can't fully understand from this side. And whatever comes next, our clients often get a glimpse before we do. They see loved ones. They talk to people who aren't visible to us. They describe presences, doorways, music, colors, light. I've seen this too many times to call it hallucination. It's something else, something tender and mysterious and deeply comforting.

But here's the part new doulas have to understand:

> **That moment wasn't about what *I* believed.**

It was about what *she* needed.

My job wasn't to validate or disprove the metaphysics of it. My job was to meet her in her reality with respect and love.

And that's what I explain to my students. Your beliefs, your religion, your spirituality, your skepticism, your cosmology, do not come into the room with you. They stay at the door. The way I see it is simple: you don't know your doctor's religion, and you shouldn't. They care for you the same either way. Your role as a doula should be no different. You are there to support *their* worldview, *their* meaning-making, *their* final experience.

When I'm in that space, my personal faith or spirituality doesn't exist. It's not about me. If my client finds peace in a prayer, we pray. If they find peace in sage and crystals, we sage. If they want silence, we sit in it. As doulas, our job is to support whatever brings them comfort, not to project what brings us ours.

Because in the end, we're not guiding people into *our* version of death. We're helping them walk toward *theirs*.

LOGISTICAL SUPPORT

This is the one everyone forgets about until it's too late, and it's the one that saves the most chaos.

Dying comes with a thousand little details. Who do we call? What happens after the last breath? Do we call 911 or hospice? Can we stay with the body? What paperwork do we need? Families panic when they realize how much they don't know.

That's why I created my **bedside binder**, a single resource that holds everything:

- End-of-life paperwork and Do Not Resuscitate (DNR) order
- Comfort care notes
- The death plan
- Hospice and emergency contacts
- Important family phone numbers
- My contact info
- Obituary drafts or letters if they've written them

When things move fast, no one wants to be digging through drawers. They grab the binder.

But the logistics also go beyond paperwork. I teach families about **legacy projects**. I always tell them: *they say each person dies two deaths, once when our body dies, and once when our name is spoken for the last time*. What kind of legacy do you want to leave behind for those you are leaving behind? That question lights people up. They start brainstorming: handwritten letters, recipe books, recorded stories, art projects, memory boxes.

These projects help people feel like they're leaving something meaningful behind, something tangible their loved ones can reach for when the grief feels too heavy.

At Death Doula School, I teach my students to remember this: logistics are love. Organization and preparation are how we make space for presence.

When all four pillars, emotional, practical, spiritual, and logistical, are working together, everything changes. The energy in the room softens. The family relaxes. The dying person breathes easier.

And that's when someone always says the same thing: "I don't know how anyone does this without you."

And I always tell them the truth: "No one should ever have to."

The Heart of the Role

While you absolutely need training to step into the role of a death doula, most of us don't find our way here because of a curriculum. We find our way here because something in us recognizes this work before we ever learn how to do it.

For me, it has always felt like something that lived inside me long before I had language for it. My nervous system was built for these moments. My energy knows how to slow a room down. When I walk into a space where someone is dying, my body doesn't panic. It settles. I don't have to force calm or remind myself how to show up. I just do. It's like some ancient part of me remembers what this threshold is, what it asks of us, and how to stand inside it without flinching.

That's not something you can teach in a weekend training. And it's not something everyone has, no matter how badly they want to help.

This work requires more than knowledge. It requires presence. Real presence. The kind that doesn't rush to fill silence, doesn't panic at discomfort, and doesn't need to fix what isn't fixable. You can learn the signs of active dying. You can memorize comfort measures. You can master care planning and logistics. But none of that matters if you can't sit in the room and *be* with what's happening.

That's the heart of the role.

I once had a client who loved Frank Sinatra more than anything. It was part of who she was. His music followed her through decades of her life, through joy and heartbreak and everything in between. One afternoon, I arrived to see her as she was laboring out of life. You could see it in her body immediately. Her face was tight. Her breathing was uneven. A low, restless sound slipped out with every exhale. She was uncomfortable and not in a way that medications alone could touch.

I didn't say a word.

I opened my phone, scrolled to her favorite Frank Sinatra song, and pressed play. I took her hand and sat beside her, quiet. No explanations. No instructions. Just presence and familiarity.

Within seconds, her body softened. The moaning stopped. Her breathing slowed. And then the smallest, faintest smile crossed her face.

That was it. No grand intervention. No heroic moment. Just knowing *who she was* and honoring it all the way to the end.

People think death doulas show up to help someone die. But that's not really what we do. We show up to help someone be fully seen. We protect their autonomy when it's easiest for it to be taken away. We remind them that they still have choices, even when those choices are small. Especially when they're small.

We are often the only person in the room who isn't afraid of death itself. Everyone else is afraid of saying the wrong thing, doing the wrong thing, hoping too much, or not hoping enough. We're the ones who can sit in the truth without trying to soften it or avoid it. We don't rush people out of grief or force them into acceptance. We let the process unfold in its own time.

And because of that, families remember death differently.

I've watched families walk away saying, "It was awful. . .but it was also beautiful." That sentence doesn't happen by accident. It happens because someone helped them slow down, stay present, and feel supported instead of overwhelmed. It happens because someone protected the space enough for meaning to exist inside the loss.

This role isn't about managing death. It's about midwifing meaning right through it.

It's about understanding that death is not a medical failure or a scheduling problem. It's a human experience. One that deserves care, attention, and reverence. When we show up this way, we don't just change the moment of death itself. We change how the living carry it forward.

Grief doesn't disappear when death is gentle, but it changes shape. It becomes less jagged. Less traumatic. Less filled with regret. Families who feel supported don't spend years replaying what they wish they'd done differently. They remember the music. The laughter. The quiet moments. The way their loved one looked peaceful at the end.

That's not an accident. That's intentional care.

At its core, being a death doula means trusting yourself enough to be still. It means knowing when to speak and when not to. It means understanding that sometimes the most powerful thing you can do is sit in a chair, hold a hand, and breathe with someone while the world changes.

It also means knowing your limits. Knowing that you can't save people from dying, and you're not meant to. This work isn't about heroics. It's about humility. About walking alongside, not leading or controlling. About honoring what is instead of fighting what isn't.

If death doulas, healthcare professionals, and families could all meet each other with mutual respect and trust, the entire experience of dying would look different. It wouldn't be cold or mechanical or rushed. It wouldn't feel like something that happens *to* people. It would feel like something people are supported through.

Death would stop being a thing we fear and start being something we understand.

Everyone deserves to be truly seen before they die. Everyone deserves a death that feels like their own. And everyone deserves to be accompanied by someone who isn't afraid to walk with them all the way to the end.

PART II

The Skills

CHAPTER 6

Communication at the End of Life

The Power of Words

Death isn't a bad word. It's just one most people haven't been taught how to say without flinching. And when we flinch, the people we're trying to support feel it immediately. They might not be able to name it, but their nervous system knows when something is being avoided. When I teach about language, the first thing I tell my students is this: *we are the ones who can change the narrative.*

Words shape how people experience reality, especially when fear is already sitting in the room. Language can tighten a space or soften it. It can escalate panic or invite grounding. It can make someone feel like they're losing control or help them feel steady enough to stay present inside what's happening.

If we're afraid to say the words death, dead, dying, then we are part of the problem. You can't dismantle a culture of fear while whispering around it. Avoidance doesn't make death gentler. It makes it lonelier. I wear the title Death Doula proudly. I say the words out loud, often. Death is not a dirty word; it's just one most people haven't been taught how to say without wincing.

When we teach people how to talk to children about death, we tell them to be honest and use clear language. We warn them not to use phrases like "passed away" or "gone to a better place" because it confuses kids and delays understanding. But for some reason, we abandon that logic when it comes to adults. As if full-grown humans need more cushioning from reality than children do.

Softening reality doesn't protect anyone. It just keeps the fear alive under the surface, where it grows and mutates. When people sense something is wrong but can't name it, their anxiety skyrockets. They feel unsteady, like the ground beneath them is shifting and no one will tell them why.

Clarity isn't cruelty. It's respect.

One of the most harmful language patterns I see around death is the way we frame illness as a battle. We say someone is "fighting cancer." We praise them for being "strong." We urge them to "keep fighting" or "never give up." And when they die, we say they "lost their battle."

I know what people mean when they say those things. They're trying to be encouraging. They're trying to convey love. But what lands is something very different.

When we frame illness as a fight, we quietly imply that survival is a matter of effort. That if someone dies, it's because they didn't fight hard enough. That strength equals staying alive. That choosing comfort over more treatment is somehow quitting or failing.

People don't die because they failed. They die because they are human. Because bodies have limits. Because death is not a moral outcome. It's a biological one. It is the one thing every single one of us is guaranteed.

Language like "lost their battle" doesn't honor someone's life. It places judgment on their death. And I see the weight of that land on families all the time. I see spouses and children replaying decisions, wondering if they should have pushed harder, tried one more thing, demanded one more treatment, as if love is measured by how much suffering you're willing to endure.

That's not love. That's fear disguised as hope.

Hope isn't always about cure. Sometimes hope is about comfort. Sometimes hope is about peace. Sometimes hope is about having the courage to choose how you want to live with the time you have left.

But we can't get there if we're afraid of honest language.

I once worked with a client whose family refused to use the word *dying*.

She was only 52, the matriarch of the family, and everyone adored her. She was the glue. The organizer. The one who remembered birthdays and kept traditions alive. The idea of life without her felt impossible, so they tried not to name what was happening to her. They avoided the word like it might make things worse if spoken.

They spoke in circles around her cancer diagnosis. Cancer without saying cancer. Decline without saying dying. They used vague language and hopeful tones, even when hope had already shifted shape.

Then one morning, she woke up different.

Her family called me early that morning, panicked, saying something felt wrong. She wasn't making sense when she spoke, and they were scared. I told them right away that this was something her medical team needed to assess immediately. They contacted her doctor, and she was sent in for evaluation and imaging that same day.

The scans confirmed what her body had already been trying to say. The cancer had progressed rapidly. One of the tumors was now pressing on the part of her brain responsible for speech and because of that she was experiencing something called *aphasia*. Her thoughts were still intact, but her ability to form words had been disrupted.

Later that day, when I arrived to support the family, I found her sitting upright in bed, eyes wide, clearly trying to communicate. Words came out jumbled and tangled. She would say, "I am. . .," and then trail off into sounds or mismatched words that didn't land where she wanted them to. You could see the frustration rising as each attempt failed.

She reached for paper and tried to write, but the letters wouldn't cooperate either. Her hands trembled. She tore the pages apart, ripping them, throwing them across the room in anger. She groaned, yelled, moaned, desperate to be understood while the people she loved stood around guessing.

"Are you hungry?"
"Do you need water?"
"Do you need your medicine?"

She shook her head again and again, tears streaming down her face, louder each time. The pain of not being understood is its own kind of suffering. It strips people of dignity in a way physical pain never can.

I watched her closely. Her breathing. The way her hand kept pressing against her chest each time she said, "I am. . .."

And suddenly it hit me.

She wasn't asking for something.

She was telling them something.

I leaned in, took her hand, and said softly, "Dying?"

The room changed instantly.

She froze, looked straight into my eyes, and nodded. Slowly. Yes.

That was it. That was the word she needed. Not because it made things worse, but because it finally made things real. She was trying to tell them what everyone already knew but no one would say. This wasn't something they could avoid anymore. This wasn't a misunderstanding. She was dying.

The yelling stopped. Her breathing steadied. The tension drained from her shoulders. The entire room softened. The kind of silence that followed wasn't heavy; it was sacred.

In that moment, she wasn't just being heard. She was being seen.

Her body responded immediately. Muscles relaxed. Breath deepened. The energy in the room shifted. I've seen this happen countless times. When truth is named, nervous systems settle. Bodies stop bracing. People stop fighting shadows and start orienting to what's actually happening.

Words have the power to trap someone inside confusion, or they can offer relief simply by voicing the truth.

I see the opposite happen too. I've watched families lose precious time because no one was willing to say the word dying. Especially in healthcare settings. Especially with cancer. There is almost always another treatment, another scan, another protocol. The system is built to do the next thing. To fight at all costs.

And sometimes, that costs everything.

People spend their final months sick from treatment, exhausted, declining faster than they would have otherwise. By the time someone finally says, "There's nothing more we can do," the body is spent and the window for meaningful planning has closed. Families are left scrambling, wishing they'd known sooner. Wishing they'd talked about wishes. Wishing they'd slowed down.

That's not because doctors don't care. It's because the system struggles with language too.

This is where my role matters. I am not part of the medical system. I'm not there to sell a treatment plan or chase a cure. I'm there to translate. To slow things down. To explain options in human language. To ask the questions no one has asked yet. To help people think about what they want, not just what can be done.

Families tell me all the time, "No one explained it like that before." Or, "I wish someone had said this sooner." Or, "Why didn't my doctor tell me I had a choice?"

Often, the information was technically there. It just wasn't delivered in a way that felt accessible, or safe, or compassionate. Tone matters just as much as truth.

You can say the right words in the wrong way and lose the entire room. You can also say very few words, delivered with care, and change everything. Language isn't just what we say. It's how we say it. When we say it. Whether our body matches our words.

I'm careful, intentional, but not timid. I speak from calm, not control. I'm never the I-know-better voice. I'm the you're-not-alone voice. The one who can say something hard without making it feel cruel.

Being a death doula means learning how to deliver truth with tenderness. Clear enough to be understood. Gentle enough to be received. Because when you do, you don't just talk about death. You teach people that it's safe to face it.

And sometimes, just as important as the words we choose, is knowing when to stop talking.

The Art of Listening

Listening is one of the most underestimated skills in death work. Everyone thinks they know how to listen, but most people are just waiting to talk. They're waiting to reassure, to explain, to fix, to redirect, to stop the discomfort.

Real listening, the kind that matters at the end of life, is something else entirely. It's not listening to respond. It's not listening to manage. It's not listening to sound helpful.

It's listening to feel.

It's listening with your whole body, your whole nervous system, your whole attention. It's listening with the understanding that what's being said is often not the most important part of the message. You're listening for meaning, for fear, for longing, for the thing hiding underneath the sentence someone feels safe enough to offer.

Sometimes it's listening to words. Sometimes it's listening to breath. Sometimes it's listening to silence. And sometimes it's listening to what *isn't* being said at all.

There's a presence that comes with that kind of listening. A stillness that quietly says, I'm here. Take your time. You don't have to perform. You don't have to explain yourself. I'm not going anywhere. That presence alone changes a room.

You're not listening for information. You're listening for truth. You're paying attention to tone, to pauses, to the way a body tightens when someone touches on something they're not ready for yet. You're watching shoulders lift, jaws clench, hands fidget. You're noticing when someone's words say one thing and their body says another.

That kind of listening isn't passive. It's an act of care. It's how we make people feel seen when words start to fail them.

I once worked with a woman I'd been supporting for close to a year. Her cancer had moved slowly at first, giving everyone time to adjust, and then all at once it didn't. By the time we reached her final weeks, her labor out was long and hard. She was tired in a way that sleep couldn't touch.

Her sister stayed close, which was beautiful, and loud.

She loved her deeply, but she processed fear out loud. She talked through it. She filled space with words and phone calls and updates and commentary. She answered texts in the room. She took calls with the TV still on. The space around the bed was rarely quiet.

Earlier in the illness, my client would snap at her. "Can you please be quiet?" she'd say. "Not right now." She wasn't subtle about it. But as her body weakened, so did her ability to advocate for herself. The requests stopped, but the need didn't.

When I arrived for visits, I could feel the tension before I even sat down. Her jaw clenched tight. Her shoulders held up around her ears. Her breath stayed shallow, like her body was bracing for impact.

I get it. I'm sensitive to noise too. Even my ears would ache sometimes from the constant stimulation.

I'd gently suggest that her sister use my visit as a chance to step out. "Go grab coffee," I'd say. "Take a walk. I've got her." And when the room finally went quiet, I wouldn't rush to fill it.

I'd sit beside her. No talking. No explaining. No fixing. Just quiet.

Within minutes, her body would soften. Her breathing would slow. The tightness around her eyes would ease. It felt like, for the first time all day, she could rest without having to manage anyone else's emotions.

Sometimes the most profound care we offer isn't what we say. It's what we remove. That's the art of listening. Learning when to speak and when not to. Knowing that silence isn't awkward, it's healing.

But listening doesn't always come easily to the people who love someone most.

I once supported a woman whose husband struggled deeply with this. He loved her. There was no question about that. But his way of coping with her dying was to surround himself with people. Lots of people.

Family. Friends. Neighbors. Church members. Old acquaintances. Anyone who would come.

Visitors were scheduled constantly. Five, ten a day sometimes. People sitting at her bedside, talking *at* her, crying, praying, telling stories, asking questions. All of it well-intentioned. All of it exhausting.

As her body declined, she needed sleep more than anything. Sleep was where she was most comfortable. It was where her pain softened and her breathing steadied. But visitors kept coming because *he* needed them.

She told him, again and again, that she didn't want visitors. She said it clearly, gently, firmly. And still, they came.

I advocated for her. Hospice advocated for her. We explained. We reframed. We tried to help him see that what comforted *him* was costing *her* the peace she deserved. He would nod. He would agree. He would tell me he'd canceled the visits. And the moment I left, the house would fill again.

It got to the point where she never wanted me to leave. Not because she needed me to *do* anything, but because when I was there, it was the only time her boundaries were respected. The only time the room stayed quiet. The only time she was allowed to simply exist in her body without an audience.

That story still sits heavy with me. Because that's what happens when listening fails. Not out of malice, but out of *unmanaged grief*. The dying person disappears under everyone else's needs.

Listening isn't just about hearing words. It's about honoring them.

I see this a lot, especially when fear is involved. People hear what they can tolerate, not what's actually being said. They respond to their own discomfort instead of the person in front of them.

At the end of life, fear rarely shows up directly. People don't always say, "I'm afraid."

They say things like:
"I just want to make sure my family is okay."
"I don't want to be a burden."
"I don't know what happens next."
"I don't want to disappear."
"I don't want to be alone when it happens."

If you're not really listening, you'll answer those with reassurance. You'll say,
"Your family will be fine."
"You're not a burden."
"It'll all be okay."

But if you *are* listening, you hear what they're actually asking.

Will my people survive this without me?
Will I be remembered?
Will I be in pain?
What comes after this?

Those questions don't need fixing. They need witnessing.

Listening is also how we honor autonomy. This is their body. Their death. Their timeline. Their choices. Even when we wouldn't make the same ones. That's not easy, especially for people coming from healthcare backgrounds where fixing is the reflex. Where silence feels like failure. Where doing nothing feels irresponsible. But in death work, listening often *replaces* fixing.

I've sat in rooms where family members needed opposite things. One person is ready to talk openly about death. Another is still clinging to cure. One needs silence. One needs noise. One wants control. One wants surrender.

My job wasn't to pick a side. It was to listen long enough to understand what each person needed, and to help create a space where no one was bulldozed.

I've watched this work beautifully too.

I once supported a woman who chose medical aid in dying. She was clear, grounded, and at peace with her decision. Her family was not. They were afraid. They were grieving. They were resistant.

We sat together and listened.

She spoke. They listened. They cried. They asked questions. They listened again.

No one tried to win. No one rushed the outcome. And eventually, even though it wasn't the choice they would have made, they understood it was *hers*. That only happened because everyone slowed down enough to really hear one another.

Listening also requires restraint. This is the part people don't talk about enough. There are moments when you know exactly what to say. When you have the words lined up, the insight ready, the explanation polished. And you choose not to speak. Because the moment isn't asking for wisdom. It's asking for space.

Choosing silence is not inaction. It's discipline. It's trusting that the room doesn't need your voice to survive. It's letting someone arrive at their own truth without interruption. It's allowing meaning to unfold instead of forcing it into a sentence.

When I listen this way, I can feel it in my body when a room settles. The air changes. The energy slows. Muscles soften. Breathing deepens. People stop bracing. That's regulation. Not because I did something impressive, but because I *stopped* doing things that were getting in the way.

I tell my students all the time: the biggest part of this work isn't talking. It's listening. We listen to stories. To regrets. To confessions people have been holding for decades. We listen to fear, anger, guilt, love. We listen to families unravel and reassemble in real time.

We become the place where things can land without being judged or redirected or cleaned up.

To be a good death doula, you have to learn how to listen with your whole being. Ears. Eyes. Heart. Body. Because sometimes, the greatest gift you can give someone at the end of their life isn't advice or comfort or answers. It's letting them feel truly heard.

Before they go.

Speaking the Unspoken

There is an unspoken rule around death: everyone knows it's coming, but no one wants to be the first to say it out loud.

Families feel it in their bones long before they admit it. Healthcare workers soften it, circle it, or bury it under language that sounds hopeful but often just delays the inevitable. And the dying person sits in the middle of it all, sensing more than anyone realizes, quietly holding the truth while everyone else pretends not to see it.

Part of our work as death doulas is to name what is already true. Not to shock. Not to strip away hope. Not to force acceptance before someone is ready. But to bring honesty into the room so peace can finally take root.

I had a client whose family hired me with one condition: they didn't want him to know I was a death doula.

They were afraid the word itself would take something from him. Afraid it would make things "real." Afraid it would break him. This was a man with stage-four stomach cancer who hadn't been able to eat for weeks, whose body was visibly failing, whose days were shrinking. Everyone around him knew what was coming. They just couldn't bring themselves to say it out loud.

I met with the family first. I asked them to imagine what it might feel like to be nearing the end of your life and have everyone tiptoe around you, pretending nothing was happening. To feel your body changing, weakening, failing you, while the people you love keep smiling and talking about the future like it's guaranteed. Eventually, with hesitation and fear, they agreed to let me be honest.

When we walked into his room together, the family hovering behind me like a shield, they said, "Dad, we brought someone we'd like you to meet."

I smiled and said, "Hi, I'm Kacie. I'm a death doula."

The room went completely still. That kind of stillness where you can feel the air shift. And then he grinned.

"Well, that's great news," he said. "Because I'm dying."

His humor broke the tension instantly. We shook hands and started talking like old friends. The family stood there stunned. After all that secrecy, all that protection, it turned out he knew. He always had. He just needed someone to acknowledge it out loud. From that moment on, everything changed.

He spoke freely about his death. Without fear. Without hesitation. We talked about what mattered most to him, how he wanted to die, how he wanted to be remembered. We planned a death that honored his humor, his dignity, his love for his family. Slowly, his loved ones began to open up too. They went from whispering the word *death* like it might summon something terrible to saying *death doula* without flinching.

But I've also seen the opposite.

I once worked with a woman with stage-four cancer who knew, deep in her body, that she was dying. Her doctors had told her there were no more treatments that would change the outcome. No more chemo. No more radiation. Her body was declining, and she could feel it every day.

Her family, however, was not ready. Not even close. They refused to talk about dying. They refused to let her talk about it. Any mention of death was shut down immediately. Instead, they clung to cures they found online. High-dose vitamin C. Ivermectin. Red light therapy. Nebulized vitamins. Injections of things with names that sounded natural and promising and completely unproven. Anything shared in a Facebook group or a comment section was fair game.

At one point, they were driving six hours to another state for experimental, nonmedical treatments they found online. She was so sick by then that she sat in the car in absolute agony, just to get there. When I asked her if this was really what she wanted, she always said yes. But her eyes told a different story. She was doing it for them.

Her body was failing. I could see it. She could feel it. But no one was willing to name it. Instead of being supported in slowing down, in resting, in choosing comfort, she was pushed to keep trying, keep fighting, keep going. These treatments didn't help her. Some of them made her sicker. None of them stopped what was coming.

By the time the truth finally broke through, there was very little time left. What that silence cost her was peace. What it cost her family was time they could have spent differently. Conversations they never had. Choices they never made. A chance to let her be held instead of dragged forward by false hope.

Silence doesn't protect people. Avoidance doesn't protect people. It just delays the pain and often multiplies it.

One of the hardest truths families struggle with is this: the dying person almost always knows before anyone else. What breaks my heart is how often they carry that knowing alone. They're afraid to tell their families because they don't want to cause pain. They don't want to be met with tears or denial or forced optimism. They don't want to hear, "You can't think like that," or "You just have to stay positive."

So they protect the people they love by playing along with the silence. But with me, they don't have to. They can say the word dying out loud. They can say, "I don't think I have much time," or "I'm tired," or "I don't want to keep doing this." And I don't flinch. I don't cry. I don't rush to reassure them with false hope. I sit with them in the truth and let it be what it is.

That's often the first place they find relief.

Telling the truth doesn't steal hope; it just changes its shape. Hope at the end of life doesn't have to mean cure. It can mean comfort. It can mean less pain. It can mean more good days than bad ones. It can mean time at home instead of in hospitals. It can mean meaningful conversations, closure, laughter, music, quiet. Hope can mean a death that feels like it belongs to them.

I've helped people admit they're tired of fighting and tired of being sick. I've helped them find the words to say, "I don't want to live the rest of my days being chemo-sick." I've sat with families as someone asked, with tears in their eyes, "Is it okay if I stop?" And I've watched the relief wash over them when they realized they didn't have to carry that question alone.

When truth is spoken with compassion, the body responds.

Speaking the unspoken isn't just about language. It's about courage. It's about choosing connection over comfort. It's about trusting that truth, delivered with love, will never break someone.

Most people spend their entire lives avoiding difficult conversations. We dodge them at work. We sidestep them in relationships. We soften them, delay them, or pretend they don't exist at all. But in death work, there is no avoiding them. We walk straight into the hardest conversations, because someone has to be willing to say the thing no one else wants to say. And they have to say it with enough compassion that the truth doesn't crush whoever hears it.

A difficult conversation, at its core, isn't really about conflict. It's about consequence. What we say and how we say it in these moments doesn't just land and disappear. It shapes grief. It shapes memory. It shapes how people remember their final days together. That's what makes these conversations so heavy. We're not just talking. We're touching the deepest parts of someone's heart, often at the most vulnerable moment of their life.

I learned this long before I ever called myself a death doula.

During the first months of COVID, when I was working as a nurse, the world felt like one long emergency. Families were locked out of facilities. Rooms were sealed. Protocols changed by the hour. Every shift, I'd scan the patient list and know, with a sick certainty, that at least one of them would not make it through the day. And when that happened, it was my job to call the family.

I still remember the first call like it happened yesterday. I dialed the number, took a breath, and realized there was no good way to say what I was about to say. How do you tell someone their loved one is dying and then tell them they can't come say goodbye because of COVID protocols?

There is no script for that. I'd say the words, and then I'd wait.

Sometimes there was silence so long I thought the call had dropped. Sometimes there was screaming. Sometimes there was sobbing so loud I had to pull the phone away from my ear. And every time, my heart broke a little more. I could picture myself on the other end of that call, and I knew I would have exploded with anger if someone told me what I was telling them.

I understood why the protocols existed. They were saving lives. But I also knew what they were stealing from people: final moments. Last touches. Goodbyes that never got to happen.

I felt trapped between compassion and compliance.

So, I did what I could. If a patient's room was on the ground floor, I'd reposition the bed so family members could stand outside and see them through the window. I'd hold up an iPad or my phone so families could FaceTime, even if all they could manage was "I love you" through tears. It wasn't enough. It would never be enough. But it was something.

At the time, I didn't have language for what I was doing. I didn't know the phrase "holding space." I just knew it felt human. I let families yell at me. Curse the rules. Cry until the line went quiet. Sometimes I cried with them.

Those calls taught me more about communication than any class ever could. They taught me that difficult conversations aren't about saying the perfect thing; *they're about being willing to stay when everything feels unbearable*. They're about not hanging up emotionally just because the conversation hurts.

That experience cracked something open in me. It was my first real lesson in what would later become my doula work: *the art of sitting with impossible emotions without trying to fix them.*

Now, when I train doulas, I tell them that difficult conversations are part of the job description. If you're doing this work well, you will have them often. You'll sit in rooms where families disagree about treatment. Where someone decides to stop chemo. Where a dying person asks, in a quiet voice, "Is it wrong that I'm tired of fighting?"

Those moments aren't failures. They're invitations.

In healthcare, difficult conversations often happen *after* something goes wrong. A complication. A sudden decline. A test result no one wanted. They're treated like emergencies, moments everyone braces for and tries to get through as quickly as possible.

In death work, these conversations *are* the work. They aren't signs that something has gone wrong. They're opportunities to talk honestly about what matters while there's still time to shape it.

I remind my students that the way you show up in these conversations sets the tone for everyone else. People mirror you. If you panic, they'll panic. If you rush, they'll rush. If you get defensive, they'll dig in.

But if you stay grounded, calm, and steady, you give everyone permission to breathe. Sometimes the most powerful thing you can do in a hard moment is to be the calmest person in the room.

When I feel tension rising, I do a quick internal check. What am I feeling? What belongs to me, and what belongs to them? If I can ground myself, I can stay present for whatever comes next. That's not about control. It's about anchoring the moment, so it doesn't spiral.

There's also a delicate balance between honesty and timing. Some people need the truth spoken plainly, without padding or metaphor. Others need it delivered slowly, like a soft landing. You learn to read the room, the dying person's readiness, the family's fear, the grief sitting just beneath the surface.

Sometimes you hold the truth gently until it can be received. Other times, you say it clearly so everyone can stop pretending. Either way, you know you've found the right moment when the room exhales.

I've been in situations where one family member hired me and another resented my presence from the start. They see "death doula" and assume their loved one has given up. Those conversations take patience. I don't argue. I don't defend my role. I listen. I show up consistently. I let my presence do the talking.

Eventually, resistance softens.

I've had people who couldn't look me in the eye at the beginning end up thanking me at the end. Trust doesn't come from convincing someone. It comes from staying.

Every difficult conversation is really about connection. When people are scared, they don't need perfect answers. They need presence. They need someone who can stand in the storm with them and not look away.

When I think back to those phone calls during COVID, I still ache for what those families lost. But I also know those moments shaped the doula I became. They taught me that communication isn't just about words. It's about how we hold someone while they're hearing them.

When we stay. When we listen. When we give people permission to feel exactly what they're feeling without trying to fix it, something shifts. A conversation that could have shattered someone becomes sacred. And when that happens, we don't just make death easier to talk about.

We amplify love.

Nonverbal Communication

Not every kind of communication needs words. In fact, at the end of life, words often fade long before connection does. People can lose speech, lose focus, lose the energy to form a sentence, and still communicate everything if you know how to pay attention.

When I think about nonverbal communication, I think about energy first.

Energy is the undercurrent that runs through every room we enter. It's the exhale someone lets out when you walk in. It's the way shoulders drop when the nervous system finally believes it's safe. It's the difference between a room that feels frantic and a room that feels steady, even when the situation is hard. You can feel it before a single word is spoken.

And here's the truth most people don't realize until they've been at a bedside: your energy speaks louder than your mouth ever could.

If you walk into a room tight, rushed, distracted, or carrying your own anxiety like a purse you refuse to put down, people feel it. The family feels it. The dying person feels it. The room responds to it. You can't fake calm. You can fake a smile, but you can't fake regulation. The body knows. That's why some of the most powerful "communication" I offer has nothing to do with what I say. It's what I embody.

A slow breath before I enter the room. A softened voice. A relaxed face. A steady presence that doesn't demand anything from anyone. I'm not here to fix what can't be fixed. I'm here to make this moment survivable. Sometimes, that's all people need.

Touch is part of nonverbal communication, but it's not the whole story. Touch can comfort, but it can also overwhelm. The trick is learning the language of the person in front of you, not the language that would comfort you.

Some people crave a hand to hold. Others do not want to be touched at all, especially as the body declines. Skin can become sensitive. Nerves can misfire. Pain can live in places you can't see. And for some people, touch can feel invasive, even if it's "gentle."

So, I teach doulas this: *presence itself* can be the simple act of touch.

Sitting close. Being steady. Breathing slowly enough that someone else's body can borrow your pace. Letting your calm become contagious. That is communication too.

Nonverbal cues will tell you everything you need to know if you're paying attention. You can see comfort in the unclenching of a jaw. Peace in the slow rise and fall of the chest. Distress in the quick dart of a hand tugging at the blanket. Anxiety in a foot that won't stop moving. A surge of panic in a change in breathing. You can watch someone's whole body relax the moment music starts or when a window opens and the room fills with fresh air. Death has its own rhythm, and so does comfort.

Sometimes the body answers questions without words.

"Is this too much?" is answered by a furrowed brow.

"Do you need quiet?" is answered by a flinch at noise.

"Are you okay with this person in the room?" is answered by the way their breath changes when that person walks in.

This is why I often say: you don't just listen with your ears. You listen with your eyes. You listen with your nervous system. You listen with your patience. You listen with your restraint.

And I learned that lesson in a deeply personal way long before I ever framed it as a "skill." My son is nonverbal and autistic, and he has taught me more about communication than any textbook ever could.

Early on, I had to unlearn the traditional way most of us are taught to communicate. Ask a question, get an answer. Make eye contact. Use words. Keep the pace moving. Explain yourself quickly. Push through the awkwardness.

That approach does not work when someone cannot communicate in the ways the world expects them to. I had to stop asking questions he couldn't answer. I had to stop expecting eye contact as proof of connection. I had to slow my own body down, because pushing for communication only made things worse. When I tried to force a moment into the shape I thought it should take, his system would push back. Not because he was being "difficult," but because he was overwhelmed.

Parenting him taught me something that now shows up in every room I walk into as a death doula: *presence matters more than progress*.

Sometimes the goal is not clarity. It's safety. Sometimes the goal is not "getting an answer." It's understanding the message without demanding words. Sometimes the most loving thing you can do is give someone extra time and not make that feel like pressure.

With my son, I learned how to listen in a different way. I watch his breathing, because it changes when he's uncomfortable. I watch his hands, because his hands tell the truth before his face does. I pay attention to meltdowns, shutdowns, stimming, scripting, pacing, body tension, and those tiny shifts that other people miss. The second he is overstimulated, I can feel it in the air. Other people might label it as "acting up" or "being bad." I know better. His nervous system is sounding an alarm. And once you learn to see that, you stop judging and you start responding. That skill translates directly to end-of-life care. When a dying person becomes nonverbal, the world around them often starts narrating them instead of listening to them. People assume. People interpret. People decide what they "must" mean.

But the body is still communicating. The room is still communicating. The energy is still communicating. Your job is to pay attention without projecting.

That's why nonverbal communication is also about consent and boundaries.

Trauma-informed care means you never assume that "comfort" looks the same for everyone. You never assume someone wants touch. You never assume someone wants visitors. You ask permission when you can. You observe when you can't. If a person's face tenses when you touch their arm, you stop. If their breath quickens when a certain family member starts talking, you notice.

If the room becomes loud and the dying person becomes restless, you don't just chalk it up to "the dying process." You ask what the environment might be doing to them. Because the environment matters. A frantic room creates a frantic body. A calm room creates a calmer body.

This is one of the reasons death doulas can be so powerful. We are not focused on tasks. We are focused on the whole atmosphere. We notice what's being communicated without words, and we respond without making it a spectacle.

Sometimes that response is simple. Lower the lights. Turn off the TV. Ask the loudest person to step out for a few minutes. Open a window. Start a playlist that feels like the person. Put a cool cloth on the forehead if it's welcomed. Offer a hand, but don't insist on it. We do small things, but they change everything.

One of my clients taught me that lesson without ever saying a word. She was in her final days, unresponsive, barely moving, making low moaning sounds that told her husband she was uncomfortable. Hospice had already adjusted her medications, but he was panicked. He looked at me like I could pull comfort out of thin air and said, "She's suffering. The meds aren't enough."

I didn't jump into action like a superhero. I didn't start talking fast. I didn't start listing possibilities. I went to her bedside and took a moment to really see her. Her brow was furrowed. Her breathing was uneven. Her jaw looked tight. Her hands kept twitching like her body couldn't settle.

So, I did what I've learned to do in every part of my life: I slowed down. I listened to what her body was saying. I turned on her favorite music, a soft piano piece she used to play while cooking. Then I picked up her favorite book and started reading out loud, not loudly, not performatively, just quietly, like the words were part of the room's rhythm.

Within seconds, her body softened. The moaning stopped. Her breathing steadied. Her forehead smoothed. She drifted into what looked like comfortable sleep. She didn't have to tell me what she needed. Her body told me. Her energy told me. The room told me.

That's the quiet magic of this work. When you stop relying on words, you start hearing everything else.

I teach doulas to look for those cues: body tension, facial expression, restlessness, changes in breath, changes in sound, a sudden shift in the atmosphere. The room can tell you as much as the person in the bed. If the room feels heavy, frantic, or unsettled, chances are the dying person feels it too. Sometimes your job is to calm the chaos without saying a single thing.

And yes, even silence communicates. Silence can say, "I'm here with you."
Silence can say, "You don't have to perform."
Silence can give someone permission to cry without being interrupted.
Silence can give someone permission to rest without being asked questions.
Silence, when it's held intentionally, becomes its own form of love.

But silence has a twin, and it's not the same thing. Silence can also be avoidance. That's where discernment comes in.

A lot of people keep a room quiet because they're afraid of what will happen if someone speaks. They're afraid of emotion. Afraid of the truth. Afraid of grief. Afraid of the moment getting "too real." That kind of silence is tense. You can feel it in the air. It's not peace; it's pressure.

Intentional silence feels different. It feels like spaciousness. It feels like permission. It feels like no one is trying to control the moment.

Nonverbal communication also means learning to trust that you don't have to earn your place in the room by talking. Some people think support means doing. Explaining. Fixing. Reassuring. Saying something wise. But at the end of life, too many words can feel like noise.

Sometimes the most respectful thing you can do is to stop trying to prove you're helpful and just be there. And this is where my son has shaped me in a way I will always be grateful for. Because being his mom forced me to stop rushing. Stop demanding clarity. Stop expecting "normal" communication.

It made me a better listener, not just to him but to everyone. It taught me that connection is not one-size-fits-all. It taught me that communication isn't always linear. It taught me that people can be deeply connected without saying a word. It taught me that if you listen with more than your ears, you will hear the truth. At the end of life, what we say often matters far less than how we show up. Your tone, your pace, your posture, your steadiness, your willingness to be quiet, all of it communicates.

Nonverbal communication reminds us that presence is its own language. Sometimes the most healing thing you can do is walk into a room, take a slow breath, soften your shoulders, sit down, and let your stillness speak for you.

Sometimes words would only get in the way. And sometimes, when someone can no longer speak, the greatest gift you can offer is to become fluent in the language that remains.

Breath. Energy. Stillness. Safety. Love, without performance.

CHAPTER 7

Navigating Fear, Faith, and Meaning

Understanding Fear

Fear is always in the room at the end of life.
Even when no one is talking about it.
Especially when no one is talking about it.

I can usually feel it before anyone names it. The energy shifts. Breathing changes. Someone starts pacing or cracking jokes that don't quite land. Someone else is asking the same question three different ways hoping for a different answer. Fear doesn't always look like tears. Sometimes it looks like control. Sometimes it looks like anger. Sometimes it looks like someone insisting they're "fine" while their body is anything but.

Fear isn't a sign that something is going wrong. It's a sign that something *real* is happening.

Most people aren't afraid of death itself. They're afraid of dying. Of the process. Of what their body will do as it starts to fail. They fear pain and suffering. They fear being uncomfortable or distressed with no way to communicate it.

They're afraid of not being able to breathe. Of choking. Of feeling trapped inside a body that no longer responds the way it used to. They fear losing control of their bowel or bladder, being embarrassed, or being exposed in front of the people they love. Others worry about being sedated, about being "out of it," about missing their final moments because their body needs medication to stay comfortable.

And almost everyone worries about losing their voice.
What if I need something and can't ask for it?
What if I'm in pain and no one notices?
What if I'm trying to say goodbye and I can't get the words out?

These fears are deeply human, and many people are hesitant to say them out loud. They worry they sound vain or dramatic or weak. But fear doesn't need permission to exist. It's already there, whether it's spoken or not. Ignoring it doesn't make it go away. It just makes it louder.

One of the most common fears I hear is about pain. People want reassurance that they won't suffer. And it's not an unreasonable fear. We've all seen the movies. We've heard the stories. We imagine death as something violent, chaotic, unbearable.

So, I slow things down. I explain what hospice care looks like. I talk about comfort. About medication. About how pain is monitored, adjusted, taken seriously. About how suffering is not something people are left alone with. Education doesn't erase fear, but it takes the edge off. It gives people something solid to hold onto instead of spiraling into worst-case scenarios.

Then there's the fear of losing control and dignity. This runs deep.

People are afraid of being talked over. Of decisions being made without them. Of becoming a body in a bed instead of a person with preferences and boundaries. They're afraid of their personality changing. Of being remembered only as "sick." Of having their final days dictated by systems instead of choice.

And the truth is, without the right support, those fears aren't unfounded.

That's why planning matters. That's why conversations matter. That's why having people around you who know your wishes matters. Because there will come a time, for most of us, when we will no longer be able to speak for ourselves. The goal isn't to maintain control forever. The goal is to transfer it intentionally, to people who will protect your dignity when you no longer can.

I've seen fear soften the moment someone realizes they still have choices. Not even the big ones, but the meaningful ones. What music plays. Who is (or isn't) in the room. When the lights are dimmed. Whether the window is open. Who speaks for them when they can't.

Control doesn't disappear all at once. And dignity isn't something that vanishes unless we let it.

Some fears aren't about death at all. They're about the people left behind. One of my clients, a woman in her early sixties, carried that kind of fear. She had a daughter in her early twenties, just the two of them against the world. Her biggest worry wasn't her illness. It was her daughter. How would she handle her mom's death? Who would remind her to eat, to sleep, to breathe when the grief hit like a wave she couldn't outrun?

We worked together for seven months. Her fear didn't disappear, but it changed shape. Together, we built a plan. We talked through who would show up for her daughter. I promised her I would be there, at the end, at the funeral, in the weeks that followed. I would check in. I would help her daughter navigate the shock and confusion that comes after losing your person.

That promise didn't fix what was happening. But it gave her something steady in the middle of the chaos. She died knowing her daughter wouldn't be alone. Sometimes easing fear isn't about solving it. It's about offering a hand to hold while someone walks straight through it.

Spousal fear comes up constantly too, especially with women. Many of my clients worry about the husband they're leaving behind. Who will manage the house? The kids? The pets? Who will steady him when everything falls apart? Women often carry entire households emotionally, and the thought of stepping away from that responsibility can feel terrifying.

And then there's the fear no one wants to admit out loud: *what happens next?*

Many people are afraid of what comes after death. Even those with strong faith sometimes panic at the end. Belief doesn't always equal certainty. I've seen people hold on fiercely, clinging to their bodies because the transition itself feels frightening. Not knowing what's on the other side can be deeply unsettling.

When that fear comes up, I don't try to convince anyone of anything. I don't preach. I don't promise answers I don't have. I share what I've witnessed. I tell them that death doesn't feel like an ending from the bedside. It feels like a shift. A softening. A transition. The air changes. The room quiets. Something moves.

For some, that brings comfort. For others, it doesn't. And that's okay. My role isn't to eliminate fear. It's to walk alongside it without flinching.

Families have their own fears too, and they're often just as heavy.

What if I don't know what to do?
What if I can't handle watching this?
What if they're in pain and I have to see it?
What if part of me wants this to be over already?

I've been in rooms where families were holding their breath. Their person had been laboring out of life for days. Everyone was exhausted. Tension thick in the air. The questions started coming. *Why is this taking so long? Is something wrong? Does it usually look like this?*

What they weren't saying was the harder truth: they were tired of watching someone they loved disappear. They felt guilty for wanting it to end. Guilty for craving relief, even if that relief came through death.

Naming that changes everything.

I'll say it gently, but clearly: you're not a monster. You love them, and watching someone die slowly is one of the hardest things a human being can do. Wanting peace for them, and for yourself, doesn't mean you want them gone. It means you're human.

You can feel the room exhale when that truth lands. Shoulders drop. Breathing deepens. Fear loosens its grip. Fear thrives in silence. It softens when it's met with honesty and calm presence.

When I sense fear before anyone names it, I ground the room first. I don't rush to speak. I let my body do the work. I slow my movements. I soften my voice. Sometimes a hand on the arm, sometimes steady eye contact, sometimes just standing there unafraid. Energy is contagious. If I'm calm, the room can find calm too.

That's what I teach doulas. Never dismiss fear. Never minimize it. Never say, "There's no reason to be afraid." There is always a reason. Meet fear with respect. Stay grounded. People mirror you. If you panic, they panic. If you can hold steady, they can breathe.

Fear at the end of life doesn't mean someone is doing death wrong. It means they care. It means they're still connected to their life, their people, their body. Our job isn't to take fear away. It's to make sure no one has to carry it alone.

Understanding fear isn't about having the perfect words. It's about having the presence to sit with the questions, even when there are no answers. Because at the end of life, people don't need certainty. They need to know it's safe enough to ask.

Meeting Faith Where It Lives

Faith and spirituality look different for everyone at the end of life. For some people, it's a Sunday ritual, a church pew, a prayer that's been whispered the same way since childhood. For others, it's the feeling of sunlight through the window, the sound of birds in the morning, the steady comfort of nature doing what nature does. For some, it's God. For others, it's energy. For plenty of people, it's not a label at all, it's just the quiet sense that there's something more happening here than what a chart can capture.

I've seen people find peace through scripture, and I've seen people find it through ocean waves and wind chimes. I've seen someone soften when a pastor walked in and started praying. I've also seen someone soften when the room finally quieted, the lights dimmed, and no one asked them to "be strong" anymore. The truth is, there isn't one right way to face death. People reach for what feels like home, and home can look like religion, or it can look like the sky.

A lot of the people who hire death doulas lean more holistic. They're drawn to energy, nature, intuition, ritual, meaning. They want a death that feels sacred without needing to look "traditional." But I've also worked with deeply religious clients who want their final days wrapped in prayer, familiar music, and spiritual structure. And I've learned something important over the years: almost everyone reaches for something bigger than themselves when the body starts to let go. Even people who swear they don't believe in an afterlife will sometimes start seeing or sensing loved ones who've already passed. It might come through dreams, through moments that feel like visitations, through a sudden calm that makes no sense on paper. Whatever you believe about that, I've witnessed it too many times to dismiss. I don't have to explain it to honor it.

One client I worked with loved the ocean more than anything. She told me, quietly, like it was a confession, that she wished she could die on the beach. She knew it wasn't realistic. She was too sick to travel and her condition was progressing quickly. So, she did the next best thing: she bought herself a small lake house with a big window facing the water. That became her version of the beach. When her final days came, we surrounded her with seashells. We played ocean sounds. We even put sunscreen on her skin so she could smell it and feel like she was there. Her hands and feet rested in trays of sand. She died facing the water, exactly how she'd wanted. That was faith for her. Not religion. Trust. The kind of trust that says, "This is how I want to meet the end of my life, and I'm allowed to make it mine."

As a doula, my beliefs don't belong in the room. They're not relevant. What matters is the dying person's framework. Their rituals. Their language. Their idea of what's next or their decision not to decide at all. Theirs is the story I'm serving. And if I can't separate my personal beliefs from my professional role, I won't be able to give my client the care they deserve. This isn't the time for me to be "right." This is the time for them to be safe. Meeting faith where it lives asks me to pay attention to what brings someone comfort and help them build around it.

Sometimes meeting faith where it lives looks simple. I've prayed with clients. I've held hands and bowed my head and let the room do what it needed to do. I've said the Shema and lit candles for Jewish families. I've stood beside families as they performed rituals I didn't fully understand but could feel the reverence in. I've burned sage and watched someone's shoulders drop like they'd finally been given permission to exhale. I've listened to drumming circles. I've nodded along to beliefs that weren't mine, not because I was pretending but because my job wasn't to debate. My job was to honor.

And sometimes meeting faith where it lives means being willing to name the hard part: faith can comfort, but it can also complicate. It can bring peace, but it can also stir up fear. Not because faith is "bad," but because humans are complicated and death has a way of pulling everything to the surface. We all have our stories about God, about worthiness, about what we've done right or wrong, about whether we'll be forgiven, about whether we chose the "correct" path. Those fears don't always show up in the beginning. They often show up when the body starts changing fast and the reality of dying stops being theoretical.

I've seen faith shift at the end of life in every possible direction. I've seen people clinging fiercely, praying constantly, asking for scripture, needing the structure to feel steady. I've also seen people abandon beliefs they held for decades, saying, "I don't think I ever really believed," or, "I can't pretend anymore." I've seen people panic because they're suddenly questioning everything.

Not in a dramatic way, but in a quiet, devastating way. A look. A pause. A sentence that lands like a stone. "What if I was wrong?" That's not a theological conversation. That's a human one. That's fear in a different outfit.

One of the most complicated faith stories I've witnessed involved a client who was raised in a Catholic home but built her adult life within the Jewish faith community after marrying her husband. On paper, everything looked settled. She had a Jewish spouse, a synagogue community, years of shared traditions woven into her everyday life.

But as she neared the end, something in her kept reaching back toward the faith of her childhood. Not because she wanted to reject the life she had built. Not because she was trying to hurt her husband or make a statement. It was deeper than that. Instinctive. As if her nervous system remembered home before her mind could explain it.

Her husband, loving her the best way he knew how, invited members of their synagogue to visit. They came with prayer, comfort, and sincere intention. And she was torn inside.

She wasn't sure what she believed anymore.

This is the kind of moment where a doula has to be very careful. It's easy to accidentally make it about the family's comfort instead of the client's. It's easy for rituals to become something done for the people standing at the bedside, not for the person in the bed. Sometimes families don't even realize they're doing it. They're reaching for what makes *them* feel less helpless. They're trying to offer what has comforted them their whole lives. They're trying to "do something," because sitting there doing nothing feels unbearable.

But the dying person gets to lead. Always.

My role in moments like that is often as a translator and protector. I might say, gently, "I can tell she's really pulling toward what feels familiar to her. Let's make space for that too." Or, "Can we ask her what she wants right now, without assuming?" Sometimes it's as minor as limiting visitors. Sometimes it's switching the kind of prayer. Sometimes it's letting silence replace constant talking. Sometimes it's bringing in the Priest as well, not as an act of rebellion but as an act of respect. And sometimes it's simply telling the family, kindly but clearly, "This is not about what we want her to believe. This is about what she needs to feel safe."

There's a firm line I hold in this work, and it's not anti-religion. It's pro-human. I respect faith deeply, but I will not support anything that overrides someone's comfort. If a ritual is soothing, beautiful, grounding, we do it. If it's agitating, confusing, or making the dying person feel pressured, we slow down and reassess. Not because anyone is wrong, but because the priority at the end of life is not performance. The priority is peace. And peace doesn't always look like what the family expected.

At the end of life, people don't need us to have answers about God. They need us to know how to hold a room where questions are heavy. They need us to stop assuming that "faith" is a single thing. Faith can mean belief, ritual, community, meaning, hope, trust, and sometimes it just means, "Please don't let me be alone." Sometimes a person is not reaching for God at all. They're reaching for love. They're reaching for something that makes the transition feel less cold.

And this is where hope comes in, because people get scared that truth and faith and hope can't coexist. They can. They absolutely can. Hope doesn't have to mean "I hope I don't die." That's not realistic. None of us is getting out of here alive, and pretending otherwise doesn't make death kinder. Hope can shift. It usually does. Hope can become: *I hope I'm comfortable. I hope my family will be okay. I hope I'm not alone. I hope I'm remembered. I hope this means something. I hope I can let go without fear.* That kind of hope isn't denial, it's courage.

Ask before you assume. Don't walk into a room and decide what "spiritual care" should look like. Listen. Learn their language. If someone wants prayer, ask what kind. If someone wants a clergy member, ask who they trust. If someone wants silence, protect it. If someone is questioning everything, don't rush to fix that. Let them be a person, not a project. And if well-meaning relatives are putting pressure on the dying person to perform belief in a certain way, be brave enough to slow the room down and bring it back to the person who matters most.

Meeting faith where it lives is not about being spiritual or religious. It's about being respectful, adaptable, and steady. It's about making room for whatever comforts the dying person, even if it's not what the family expected, even if it looks messy, even if it changes week to week. Because faith shifts. People evolve. Dying doesn't create new people, it reveals who they've always been under the roles, expectations, and performances. What's left is raw honesty, and that includes faith, or the lack of it, or the uncertainty in between.

If faith gives someone a way to let go, I will help hold that thread. If faith is tangled up with fear, I will sit in that too, and I will not rush them. If someone's "faith" is nature, energy, music, family, the rhythm of waves through a window, I will treat that with the same respect as any prayer.

What matters most at the end of life isn't whether someone believed the "right" thing. What matters is whether they felt safe enough to be honest about what they believe now. And if I can help create that safety, then I'm doing my job.

The Search for Meaning

At the end of life, people don't suddenly turn into philosophers. They don't start quoting poetry or trying to crack the code of the universe. They don't sit around asking big, abstract questions just for the sake of it. What they want to talk about is their life. The real one. The messy one. The one that happened.

They talk about love. About the people who mattered. About the relationships that shaped them, healed them, broke them, or followed them their entire lives. They talk about things they're proud of and moments that still make them smile, even when smiling feels unexpected. They talk about memories that feel warm, familiar, safe. Meaning, at the end of life, doesn't arrive as some grand revelation. It shows up quietly, wrapped inside ordinary moments and stories that remind people who they've been.

And woven into those stories, almost inevitably, are the ones that still ache.

Most people don't lead with regret. Not right away. Regret tends to hide underneath other emotions first. It disguises itself as frustration, as sadness, as restlessness. Sometimes it leaks out sideways, as irritability or anger. It takes time and trust before someone finally says the thing that's been sitting heavy in their chest for years. But when they do, when the "I wish I had. . ." finally comes out, something shifts. Their breathing changes. Their shoulders drop. It's like the body knows it can finally put something down.

That's one of the quiet miracles of this work. The way a conversation can lift emotional weight just as effectively as medication can ease physical pain. Something most people don't realize is that when people are allowed to tell the truth about their lives without being rushed, corrected, or reframed, they soften. They die calmer. Lighter. More at peace.

I once worked with a man in his late sixties, a retired truck driver with a sharp sense of humor and a deep loyalty to black coffee and bad diner food. Early on, he told me, "I don't need to talk about my feelings. I'm fine." This, of course, is what people say when they do need to talk about their feelings because they are very much not fine.

But, knowing his kind, I didn't push. We talked about football. About the terrible hospital food. About how the one nurse definitely had a crush on the other nurse. I let him lead the conversation wherever he wanted it to go. And then one afternoon, out of nowhere, he said, "You know what I keep thinking about? That time I missed my daughter's graduation."

Just like that, the wall cracked.

He told me about a long haul he couldn't get out of, about promising her he'd make it back in time, about a snowstorm that delayed him for days. He never forgave himself, even though she had. "She told me it was fine," he said. "But it wasn't fine to me."

I didn't try to fix it. I didn't offer him a lesson about forgiveness or tell him everything happens for a reason. I just sat with him while he said it out loud. When he was done, he exhaled, a real exhale, like he'd been holding that story in his body for 30 years.

That's what the search for meaning usually looks like. It isn't about answers. It's about unburdening.

Sometimes meaning shows up more urgently. Not because someone wants to reflect, but because something breaks the illusion that there's still plenty of time. I've worked with people who've faced serious illness more than once. They go through treatment, recover, rebuild their lives, and then it comes back. And then it comes back again. By the time they end up working with me, they aren't asking hopeful questions anymore. They're tired. They're confused. And eventually, they ask the question they've been circling for years.

Why me? Why does this keep happening to my body? Why can't it just leave me alone?

There's no good answer to that. I don't have one. I wish I did.

I don't try to answer it. I sit with them in the question. I let them say it as many times as they need to. I let them be angry about it. Or sad. Or exhausted. Sometimes the most honest thing you can say is, "I don't know." People don't need explanations in those moments. They need someone who isn't afraid of their uncertainty.

When people start talking about regret, what they're usually grieving isn't one specific event. It's time. The way they assumed there would always be more of it. They talk about working too much. About waiting too long. About thinking they'd get around to the important stuff later. Later becomes a very loud word at the end of life.

Meaning also shows up in quieter ways. I once worked with a woman whose life looked unremarkable on paper. No big achievements. No dramatic stories. She talked mostly about caring for people, her kids, her neighbors, her aging parents. At one point she looked at me and said, almost apologetically, "I don't think I did anything special."

But as she talked, it became clear that she had been the steady presence in a lot of lives. The one people called when things fell apart. The one who showed up. The meaning of her life wasn't a headline. It was accumulation. Love, given consistently, over time.

Not everyone wants to go deep every day. And that's okay. Some days, meaning looks like talking about a favorite TV show or arguing about whether pineapple belongs on pizza. Humor matters. Normalcy matters. If laughing about something stupid helps someone feel human again, then that matters too. Meaning hides there as well.

When people have their practical plans in place, their care preferences, their logistics, their wishes clearly known, it frees up space for reflection instead of panic. That's when stories start to come out naturally. "Did I ever tell you about the time. . ." becomes an invitation. A way of remembering themselves as more than a diagnosis.

There are things that get in the way of meaning, though. Platitudes. Forced optimism. Being told to "stay positive" or "keep fighting." Those phrases shut people down. They rush them past honesty and into performance. Meaning can't survive where truth isn't allowed.

I don't try to pull meaning out of people. I don't guide them toward it. I make space for it and let it arrive on its own, in whatever form it takes. Sometimes it's a heavy conversation. Sometimes it's a memory. Sometimes it's just sitting quietly together while someone remembers who they've been.

I often ask, "What's top of mind for you today?"
Not because I need a deep answer, but because it gives people permission to go wherever their heart, and head already is.

Meaning doesn't come from perfect endings. It comes from presence. From being heard. From being allowed to tell your story without someone rushing to interpret it.

At the end of life, meaning is less about answers and more about presence. Less about figuring it out and more about being witnessed. Sometimes the most sacred thing you can do is sit with someone while they remember their life, not to define it, not to judge it, but to honor that it was lived.

Something happens when people begin to approach the end of their lives. The edges of belief soften. The lines that once felt solid start to blur. The rules, the rituals, the certainty people have leaned on for decades can suddenly feel too small to hold what they're experiencing now.

For some people, belief tightens. They cling harder than ever to the faith that has carried them through their lives. Prayer becomes constant. Rituals become anchors. Familiar words are repeated like lifelines. For others, belief loosens. Questions rise. Doubts surface. And sometimes, quietly, people realize that what they've believed for years may not actually be theirs.

I've seen both. Often in the same family. Sometimes in the same room.

I once worked with a woman whose religion didn't allow for talk of spirits, visions, or the presence of the dead. She had followed those teachings her entire life. Faith was her structure. It gave her rules, answers, and a sense of order in the world. But as she moved closer to death, something shifted. She began seeing her parents, her brother, and her childhood best friend—people who had died long before her. She described them with clarity and certainty, not confusion. "They're here," she told me. "They've come to walk me home."

Her family tried to correct her at first. They told her the medications were causing hallucinations. That she was confused. That she shouldn't say things like that. But she wasn't confused. In fact, she was clearer than I had ever seen her. Her voice was steady. Her body was calm. One afternoon she looked at me and said, "I've believed a lot of things in my life, but I've never known anything this surely."

In those final days, she didn't reject her faith in anger or rebellion. There was no dramatic unraveling. She simply released it. Quietly. Gently. She no longer needed someone else's framework to explain what she was experiencing. She trusted her own knowing. And the peace in the room was undeniable. Her breathing slowed. Her face softened. There was no fear in her eyes. Just readiness.

That's something death does. It strips belief down to its essence. It removes performance. What's left is experience.

Not everyone moves toward peace so easily.

I've also sat with people whose beliefs began to scare them as the end drew closer. People who had lived their entire lives certain of what came next, only to find that certainty cracking under the weight of dying. I've heard the questions whispered late at night, when the room is quiet and the fear finally surfaces. What if I was wrong? What if I didn't believe the right way? What if this isn't enough?

Those moments aren't loud. They're fragile. A tightening in the chest. Restless hands. Eyes searching for reassurance that no one can honestly give. This is where belief stops being abstract and becomes deeply personal. It's no longer about doctrine or rules. It's about fear. And fear doesn't care how long you've believed something. It shows up anyway.

When that happens, I don't rush to correct it or soothe it away. I don't argue someone out of what they're feeling. I don't reach for theology or platitudes. I've learned that certainty is rarely what people need in those moments. What they need is permission to not know.

When someone looks at me and asks, "What happens next?" I don't pretend I have the answer. I tell them the truth. I tell them I've sat bedside with hundreds of people as they've died. I tell them that the energy in the room at the moment of transition is always the same. It's calm. It's gentle. It's not scary. I tell them I've never felt panic in those moments, only a deep stillness, like something settling into place. That's not proof of anything. But it's real. And sometimes that's enough.

Families don't always handle belief shifts easily.

I once worked with a young woman in her twenties whose body was failing far sooner than anyone expected. As she neared the end, she began seeing things she couldn't explain—loved ones, energies, presences that brought her comfort. She spoke about them calmly, almost casually. But her family struggled. What she was describing didn't fit within the framework of the religion she had been raised in. They wanted to believe her, but they were torn between trusting her experience and honoring the teachings they'd always known.

The room felt tense in those moments. You could feel the discomfort hovering in the air. No one wanted to say the wrong thing. No one wanted to invalidate her, but no one knew how to reconcile what she was experiencing with what they believed. I didn't try to explain it. I didn't label it. I didn't spiritualize it or medicalize it. I simply honored her experience as hers. And slowly, the tension eased. Not because the questions were answered, but because no one was being told they were wrong.

That's one of the quiet lines I hold firmly in this work: I will never argue someone out of what they're experiencing at the end of life, even if it contradicts their lifelong beliefs, even if it scares the family, even if it doesn't make logical sense, even if it can't be explained medically. Belief doesn't always fade at the end of life. Sometimes it expands. Sometimes people who were rigid in their thinking soften.

Others who never believed in anything beyond what they could see begin talking about connection in ways they never did before. They start saying things like, "I don't know what's next, but I don't think it's nothing." Or, "I think this is going to be okay."

And sometimes belief simply changes shape. It becomes less about answers and more about trust. Trust in the process. Trust in the people around them. Trust that whatever comes next won't be worse than what they're leaving behind.

When people spiral because they want certainty—because not knowing feels unbearable—I bring them back to the moment they're in. I slow my voice. I ground the room. I remind them that they're not dying all at once. They're here, now. Breathing. Held. Safe. And when fear settles, even just a little, you can see it in their bodies. Their shoulders drop. Their jaw softens. Their breathing deepens. The grasping eases.

Sometimes people die holding tightly to what they've always believed. Sometimes they die having let it all go. And sometimes they die somewhere in between, suspended in wonder, uncertainty, and trust.

And honestly, that's enough.

There are questions in this work that never get answered. Not because we aren't asking them hard enough, or because we're missing some secret knowledge, but because they simply aren't meant to be answered while we're still here.

What happens after death?
Where does the energy go?
Do they see us again?

I don't know. And what surprises people most is how deeply at peace I am with that.

I've always been this way. Long before I became a death doula, long before I sat at hundreds of bedsides, I understood death as something expected. Not welcome, not easy, but natural. We are born, we live, and we die. That arc has never felt cruel to me. It has always felt honest. Even when people I love die, I grieve their absence, but I'm not shaken by the fact of their death. It doesn't fracture my understanding of the world. It fits.

Maybe that's just how I'm wired. Maybe it's something older than logic. I've had a medium tell me my soul has been here many times before, that this isn't my first round, and maybe that's true. Maybe that's why death feels familiar to me in a way it doesn't to most people. I don't need to know if that's right to feel the comfort of it. I just know that when death shows up, my body doesn't recoil. It recognizes it.

Families don't always know what to do with that.

They want answers. They want certainty. They want someone to tell them what comes next so they can hold onto something solid while everything else is falling apart. And sometimes they look at me like I'm withholding something when I say, "I don't know."

But what I've learned is that certainty isn't what most people are asking for. What they're asking is, "Am I going to be alone in this?" And that question, I can answer.

I've watched families relax when they realize I'm not going to feed them platitudes. I'm not going to invent a story about heaven or timelines or guarantees. I'm not going to say, "Everything happens for a reason," or, "They'll be watching over you," unless that belief already belongs to them. What I will say is this: *I'm here. I'm not afraid. And you don't have to carry this by yourself.* I once worked with a woman who was terrified of what would happen after she died. Her body was exhausted. Her breathing was shallow. Everything about her looked ready to let go, except her fear. She hovered in that space for days. Then weeks. Her family sat by helplessly, watching her suffer, watching her linger, unable to understand why she couldn't release.

I could feel it in the room. She wasn't holding on because she loved her life too much to leave it. She was holding on because she was afraid of what came next.

One afternoon, I leaned close to her. I wasn't nervous. I wasn't unsure. I didn't plan what I was going to say. It wasn't rehearsed or symbolic. It was instinctive, like something in me knew exactly what she needed. I told her the truth.

I told her I knew she was scared. I told her I knew she didn't know what was next. And then I told her something else, something that mattered more than any answer: that what was happening here wasn't meant for her anymore. Her body couldn't carry her soul. It was tired. It was failing her. And whatever came next had to be gentler than this.

I told her it was a beautiful day outside. The kind of day made for transition. I promised her she wasn't alone. And then I said, "Let's do this together."

I walked out of her room. I went down the hallway and opened the front door. I stood in the sunlight and called her name. I told her to look at how beautiful it was. I told her it was okay to come with me.

Then I left.

Two minutes later, her husband called. She had taken her last breath.

She didn't need to know *where* she was going. She just needed permission to *go*.

That moment taught me something I now carry into every room: peace doesn't come from answers. It comes from trust. From knowing you're not being abandoned in the not-knowing.

When I teach doulas, I'm honest about this part of the work. I tell them there will be moments when clients or families look at them and beg, "Please just tell me what happens next." And I tell them it's okay to say, "I don't know." In fact, it's often the most ethical thing you can say.

Our power is not in certainty. It's in presence. It's in staying when things stop making sense. It's in not rushing people toward closure or meaning or acceptance. It's in resisting the urge to fill silence with explanations just so *we* feel useful.

I don't believe death is random or cruel. I don't believe we're meant to understand everything. I don't believe answers are required for peace. I do believe that love carries people farther than explanations ever could.

Walking without answers means trusting the moment instead of controlling it. It means allowing mystery to exist without trying to tame it. It means understanding that saying "I don't know" doesn't make you weak; it makes you honest.

When fear creeps in, when families press for certainty, when you catch yourself wishing you could explain the unexplainable, pause. Take a breath. Ground yourself. Remember that your presence matters more than your words ever will. Because none of us walks through death with a map. But none of us has to walk it alone.

CHAPTER 8

Planning and Preparation

Why Planning Matters

People avoid end-of-life planning for the same reason they avoid going to the dentist or cleaning out the junk drawer. It feels uncomfortable. Inconvenient. Easier to ignore than deal with. Most people assume they'll get to it later, when things are calmer, when there's more time, when it feels more appropriate to talk about dying.

But the truth is, there is rarely a perfect time. And later is a luxury not everyone gets.

Planning for the end of life isn't about being morbid or pessimistic. It's about being realistic. It's about acknowledging that death is not a failure or an anomaly; it's the natural conclusion of a human life. And when we plan for it, we aren't giving up hope. We're reclaiming power.

When I walk clients through their planning process, the biggest emotional shift I see isn't fear. It's relief. Then calm. Then something that surprises them most of all: control. It's like watching someone exhale for the first time in months, sometimes for the first time since their diagnosis. Their shoulders drop. Their voice softens. The frantic edge that's been living under the surface finally quiets.

Once people realize how much of their death they can influence, how their environment looks, who's in the room, who isn't, what kind of care they receive, what they want their final days to feel like, they begin to reclaim ownership of an experience most people assume will simply happen to them. For so many, this is the first time in a long time they've felt true bodily autonomy.

Planning helps dissolve fear because it turns the unknown into something visible. Something nameable. Something manageable. It takes the abstract terror of "someday" and brings it into the present moment, where choices can still be made. And the more we talk about it, the less power it has over us.

Of course, I get pushback all the time.

"We'll do that later."
"It's too soon."
"I'm not ready to talk about that yet."

My answer never changes. It's never too soon.

I've seen what happens when people wait. I've seen the cost of silence and avoidance. As a nurse, and now as a death doula, I've watched families unravel at the bedside because nothing was decided ahead of time. I've seen siblings screaming at each other over feeding tubes and ventilators while their parent was actively dying. I've seen partners paralyzed by guilt, terrified of making the wrong choice because they didn't know what their person would have wanted.

I've seen people who were very clear, verbally, about wanting a Do Not Resuscitate order, only to have their wishes overturned at the last minute because the paperwork wasn't in place and their power of attorney panicked. I've watched people suffer through aggressive medical interventions they never wanted because they lost the ability to speak for themselves before choosing who would speak for them. When no healthcare proxy is designated, decisions default to whoever is next in line, whether they are emotionally capable, informed, or aligned with the person's values or not.

I've seen people taken advantage of. I've seen people treated poorly. I've seen people spend their final weeks or months in facilities they hated because no one planned for how they could be supported at home. I've done CPR on a 106-year-old woman with terminal cancer because her power of attorney refused to sign a DNR. I had to break nearly every rib beneath my hands to restart her heart, just so she could live 12 more hours in agony with a crushed chest.

That is what happens when there is no plan.

End-of-life planning is not the conversation you have after everything falls apart. *It's the conversation that prevents it from falling apart in the first place.*

Most people think end-of-life planning is about paperwork. Wills. Finances. Lawyers. And yes, those things matter. But that's only part of the picture. What people rarely think about is themselves. Their body. Their comfort. Their dignity.

When I start asking clients questions about what they want for themselves, how they want their days to feel, where they want to be, who they want nearby, they're often caught off guard. They've planned meticulously for their belongings but never considered that they might get to plan their dying.

Once we move beyond documents and into what I call the death plan, people are shocked by how much autonomy they have. They didn't know they could choose the lighting in the room or whether they want music or silence. They didn't know they could decide who is present and, just as importantly, who is not. Many people carry complicated family dynamics, and being clear about boundaries at the end of life is an act of self-protection, not cruelty.

They didn't know they could plan for sunlight through a window instead of harsh overhead lights, for LED candles instead of sterile hospital glare, for stories and laughter instead of constant monitoring. They didn't realize they could make their final days feel gentle, familiar, and human.

That realization changes everything. The emotional shift is visible. Conversations become less tense. Bodies soften. Sleep improves. People who were once nervous and guarded start looking forward to our meetings instead of dreading them. Their questions become thoughtful instead of frantic. They stop spiraling and start settling.

And planning doesn't just change things for the person who is dying. It is one of the greatest gifts you can give the people you leave behind.

When plans are clear and communicated, families grieve without second-guessing. They don't spend months replaying decisions in their minds, wondering if they did the right thing. They don't fracture under the weight of "what if." Siblings are far less likely to fight. Partners are less likely to carry guilt. There is clarity where there would have been chaos.

This is why communication matters just as much as documentation.

You can have every form completed and every wish written down, but if your loved ones don't know the plan, conflict will still find its way in. That's why, as a death doula, I don't just help people plan. I help them talk. I facilitate conversations with partners, children, and families so everyone is on the same page before things get hard. When those conversations happen early, people show up with love instead of fear.

End-of-life planning doesn't erase grief. It clears a path through it.

It transforms panic into purpose and confusion into clarity. It ensures that when someone can no longer speak for themselves, their voice is still heard. Their dignity is still protected. Their wishes are still honored.

End-of-life planning is really about peace, not paperwork. It's about love, not logistics. It's about making sure that when the time comes, the people you care about most are free to simply be present, instead of being forced to make impossible decisions in the middle of heartbreak.

That's why planning matters. It gives people back their voice, their peace, and their power, exactly when they need it most.

The Conversations No One Wants to Have

Planning is the easy part. Talking about it is what breaks people open.

As long as things stay theoretical, people can keep their footing. Planning lives in the abstract, in ideas, not emotions. It's easier to stay composed when decisions feel distant and hypothetical, when no one has to picture themselves saying the words out loud yet. But the moment we start talking about saying it out loud, to their spouse, their kids, their parents, that's when the room shifts.

Shoulders tense. Eyes dart. Someone suddenly needs to use the bathroom. Jokes get made. Silence stretches longer than it should. End-of-life conversations carry weight, and everyone feels it, whether they admit it or not.

Every family has that one topic that makes their stomach drop. The one they hope someone else will bring up first.

For some families, it's medical decisions. CPR. Feeding tubes. Dialysis. Ventilators. Words that sound clinical until you imagine them attached to someone you love. For others, it's hospice. That single word can make people flinch, like saying it out loud might make death move faster, as if hospice itself is a curse rather than a support. And then there are families who can handle all the medical talk just fine but completely fall apart when it's time to discuss funeral plans. That's when the loss becomes real. That's when imagining *someday* turns into imagining *soon*.

I had one client who avoided end-of-life planning entirely because she didn't feel sick enough yet. Every time we circled back to it, she reassured herself she had more time. Her symptoms were manageable. Her mind was clear. She wasn't ready to look at what was ahead. And in many ways, I understood that instinct. No one wants to sit with mortality before they feel forced to.

Then one day, everything changed.

Her condition progressed quickly. Cognition declined. Decisions had to be made in crisis. Nothing was written down. Nothing had been communicated. What followed was panic, not because she was dying but because no one knew what to do *for* her. Her family wasn't grieving yet; they were scrambling. They were terrified of getting it wrong. They were arguing not because they disagreed on values, but because they had never been given clarity.

Most people think avoiding these conversations is a kindness. They believe they're protecting themselves, or their loved one, from pain. What they're really doing is pushing that pain forward, into a moment when everyone is already overwhelmed, exhausted, and afraid.

This is why I come back to the same truth over and over again: you have to choose your *hard*.

Having these conversations now is hard. Sitting down and naming what might happen is uncomfortable. It makes things feel real. It strips away the illusion of control. But not having them is even harder. Later down the road when decisions are rushed, emotions are raw, and everyone is afraid of making the wrong call with no guidance to lean on.

People avoid these talks not because they don't care. They avoid them because they care deeply. They're afraid of upsetting the dying person. Afraid of saying the wrong thing. Afraid of being blamed later. Afraid of disagreeing and not being able to fix it. Afraid that once it's spoken, it can't be unsaid. Afraid that acknowledging death somehow accelerates it.

And sometimes, they're afraid that talking about death will somehow invite it in. It won't. Talking about death doesn't make it happen sooner. It just makes it less chaotic when it does.

This is one of the most important pieces of education I offer families. Death does not need your permission to arrive. Silence doesn't delay it. Avoidance doesn't protect anyone. What silence and avoidance do is strip people of the chance to move through the end together with intention. When I facilitate these conversations, my role isn't to force comfort or consensus. It's to create clarity.

When things get tense among families, which will always happen, I'm the calm in the storm. I stay neutral. I don't take sides. I slow people down when emotions start colliding. I translate when language gets confusing. I redirect when conversations spiral into fear-based hypotheticals. And when things drift off course, I bring everyone back to the same place: we are here because we love this person and want their final chapter to be as gentle as possible. That reminder alone can change everything.

I've had families where everyone was holding their breath, waiting for someone else to speak first. Once one honest sentence landed, "I'm scared," or "I don't know what to do," or "I don't want them to suffer," the entire room softened. Not because the situation improved, but because the truth finally had air. Once truth enters the room, people stop posturing and start connecting.

After the conversation happens, there's often a strange mix of emotions. Relief, yes, but also sadness. Talking about what the end may look like makes loss feel closer. It collapses distance. It removes denial. And that can feel heavy.

But once it's out in the open, something shifts. People sleep better. Questions become more thoughtful instead of frantic. Families start working together instead of bracing for impact. Decision-making becomes steadier. The energy in the room changes. There is less panic and more presence.

Avoidance dissolves. Presence arrives.

One of the most misunderstood parts of this work is that these conversations aren't about controlling death. They're about controlling chaos. They reduce second-guessing. They reduce guilt. They reduce the "what ifs" that haunt people long after someone is gone.

When planning is communicated, not just completed, but shared, families move through the end together instead of fracturing under the weight of unspoken expectations. Drama loses oxygen. Even disagreement becomes easier to navigate when the person at the center has been heard.

Silence doesn't spare people. It just makes them unprepared. That's why these conversations matter. Not because they're easy. Not because they feel good. But because they create space for love to show up when it matters most, without chaos, without confusion, without regret.

Talking about what no one wants to talk about doesn't summon death. It just makes room for peace.

End-of-Life Planning

End-of-life planning is not glamorous, but it is one of the most important things you will ever do. It is where clarity meets compassion, not just for the person who is dying but for everyone who will be left to navigate what happens after. When it is done well, it rarely gets noticed. Things simply unfold with less panic, less confusion, and less regret.

When I talk about end-of-life planning, I am talking about everything that helps bring order to chaos. Advance directives. Do not resuscitate orders. Healthcare power of attorney. Financial power of attorney. Funeral planning. Financial planning. Conversations about hospice. Even Swedish death cleaning. Anything that reduces uncertainty and protects a person from becoming the center of crisis during their most vulnerable moments.

But it is important to be clear about the role of the death doula in this process. Death doulas do not complete legal or financial paperwork for clients. We are not estate attorneys, funeral directors, or financial planners. Those roles matter deeply, and those professionals are essential. Our role lives alongside theirs. We are the ones checking in, asking questions, and making sure those pieces exist and are current. When something has not been done, we help connect clients with the right professionals and then support the conversations that bring those plans to life. We also help them to understand the planning, what needs to be thought of and why it needs to be done.

End-of-life planning touches on far more than people realize. Working with an **estate attorney** is not just about drafting a will. It is about choosing a healthcare power of attorney who truly understands your values. It is about naming who will make decisions if you cannot speak for yourself. It is about protecting the people you love from probate court when that can be avoided. It is about ensuring that the person you trust is legally empowered to act, not just emotionally willing.

Financial planning matters just as much, and it is something people benefit from starting far earlier than they think. Ideally, this begins in your twenties or thirties, long before illness enters the picture. Financially planning for the end of your life ensures you get choices. Do you want to die at home if that is possible? Do you want professional caregivers involved, or are you expecting family to step into that role? Many people do not realize that full-time caregiving is incredibly expensive. In-home care can cost several thousand dollars a month, and long-term care facilities can cost anywhere from $8,000–$10,000 per month or more. When there is no financial plan in place, those decisions are no longer choices. They become burdens placed on families who may already be overwhelmed.

Some people know they would prefer to be cared for in a long-term care facility rather than at home. Others feel strongly about remaining in familiar surroundings. There is no right answer, but there is a need to think about it. These preferences affect finances, caregiving arrangements, and family dynamics long before the end arrives.

Funeral planning is another area that has changed dramatically over the last decade. Many people still imagine funerals as limited to burial or cremation, but the options today are far broader and more personal. Green burials, shrouding, human composting, aquamation, burial at sea, being incorporated into a coral reef, ashes turned into diamonds or Parting Stones, even companies that preserve tattoos after death. These are not fringe ideas anymore. They are real options that allow people to align their death with their values.

Having these conversations early opens the door for choice rather than default. It also helps families avoid unnecessary pressure and cost. Something as simple as knowing you can purchase an urn online for a fraction of what a funeral home may charge can make a meaningful difference. Planning does not mean stripping death of meaning. It means reclaiming it.

We are the bridge between "I will get around to it someday" and "this is handled."

That distinction matters, because many people assume end-of-life planning is complete simply because something was done at some point in the past. I see this often. Someone sat down with an estate attorney 20 years ago. They created a will. They named a power of attorney. They walked away feeling responsible and prepared. And for a long time, that may have been true.

But life changes.

Marriages shift. Divorces happen. Children grow up. Relationships evolve. Estrangements form. Diagnoses appear. What felt solid decades ago may no longer reflect the reality of someone's life or wishes today. An old plan can create just as much chaos as no plan at all if it has not been reviewed and updated.

False confidence is one of the most dangerous forms of unpreparedness.

I also see families who rely heavily on verbal wishes. "I have told them what I want," people will say. "They know." And maybe they do. But verbal wishes are not legally binding. Under stress, memory changes. Emotions complicate things. People hear what they want to hear. Without documentation, even the most loving families can find themselves in conflict, each person convinced they are honoring the same person in different ways.

There is also a common assumption that hospice will simply handle everything. Hospice does incredible work, but they cannot override legal authority, and they cannot fill in gaps that were never addressed. Hospice supports care. They do not replace planning.

End-of-life planning is not just about documents. It is about communication. This is where the work gets harder and where people are most likely to stall. Planning makes things real. It forces people to confront death directly, often for the first time. For someone who already carries a general fear of death, even a simple conversation can feel monumental. It is much easier to avoid it, to tell yourself there is time, to promise yourself you will deal with it later. Until later never comes.

I worked with a client in her early fifties who had terminal cancer. She was thoughtful, clear-headed, and deeply connected to her adult son. She wanted him to be her healthcare power of attorney. The complication was that she was still legally married to her estranged husband, a man who had been abusive toward her.

We talked many times about the importance of meeting with an estate attorney. I connected her with a trusted colleague who reached out repeatedly to schedule an appointment. Each time, my client said she would do it next week. She felt okay. She was managing. She was not ready to face it head-on.

Then one morning, everything changed. She woke up confused and disoriented. Her son rushed her to the hospital, and she never returned home. She never regained her cognition. Because the legal paperwork had not been completed, her estranged husband automatically became her medical decision-maker. He took over all decisions. Her son, the person she trusted most, had no legal authority to act on her behalf. All because a few documents were not completed in time.

I have also seen the other side of this story. Clients who completed their planning early, revisited it when life changed, and spoke openly with their families about their wishes. By the time I entered their care, there was room to breathe. They were not scrambling or second-guessing. They were living. Their deaths unfolded with intention, surrounded by love, without panic or power struggles.

End-of-life planning is not about controlling death. It is about preserving autonomy. It gives people the ability to make choices about how they live all the way up to their last moment. When planning is done thoughtfully, fear often softens. People become more present. Families stop hovering and start connecting. The energy in the room shifts from frantic to intentional.

This is where death planning intersects with something deeper.

Sensory-Friendly Death Plan

A death plan is different from legal paperwork. Much like a birth plan, it is about the experience rather than the legality. It considers the environment, the senses, the lighting, the sounds, who should be present and who should not. It asks what would make someone feel calm, safe, comfortable, or even held during their final days. It invites intention into a space that is often treated as purely medical.

When I talk about creating a death plan, I always say it is just like a birth plan, only on the opposite end of life. Where a birth plan focuses on how you want to come into the world, a death plan focuses on how you want to leave it. It is about bringing intention, comfort, and choice into one of the most vulnerable and sacred experiences we will ever have: dying.

Most people assume the end of life is something that simply happens to them, that they will lose agency once their body begins to fail. But the truth is that there is far more within their control than they realize. Once the legal and logistical planning is handled, the advance directives, the power of attorney, the funeral arrangements, we move into something deeper and far more personal: the lived experience of dying.

Now we get to create what I call a sensory-friendly death plan. Not because everyone wants something elaborate or beautiful, but because everyone deserves to feel safe, respected, and at ease in their final days. Dying is an intensely sensory experience. The nervous system is heightened. Sounds feel louder. Light can feel harsh. Touch can feel soothing or overwhelming. Every detail matters more than people expect.

So, I start by asking questions.

What sounds make your nervous system feel calm? Music? Laughter? The quiet hum of a room filled with people you love? The sound of ocean waves or birds outside the window? Or maybe nothing at all. Some people want sound. Others want silence. All are valid.

What scents bring you peace? Lavender? Fresh coffee? Chocolate chip cookies baking in the oven? Because if it is cookies, I will absolutely be in the kitchen baking. The sense of smell is powerful. It can ground someone, calm them, and bring them back to moments of safety and joy.

What fabrics make you feel safe and comfortable? Soft blankets or crisp sheets? A familiar sweater? Or nothing at all. Some people crave comfort through touch. Others feel overwhelmed by it. Dying is intimate, and the body's needs deserve to be honored.

What can we surround you with that would make you feel the calmest? Photos of your family? A slideshow of favorite places projected onto the ceiling? What kind of lighting feels the safest to you? Natural light pouring through a window? Overhead lighting? Or just a few lamps?

We talk about all of it.

Because dying is intimate. It is vulnerable. And in that way, it mirrors birth. So, we also talk about who is allowed in the room, and who is not. Who brings peace. Who brings chaos. Who feels grounding. Who feels draining. Some people want a room full of loved ones, laughter, storytelling, and reminiscing. Others want only one or two trusted people. Some want privacy so deep they prefer to die alone.

There is no wrong way to want this.

I have worked with clients who wanted to be read to from a children's book their mother once read to them, the familiar rhythm of the story carrying them back to a place of safety. I have worked with parents who were dying and wanted to be surrounded by photos of their children, reminders of the life they built and the love they poured into the world. I have worked with people who wanted minimal visitors, limited stimulation, and long stretches of quiet.

The death plan makes room for all of it.

It also creates clarity when emotions run high. Families often want what they think is best. Sometimes that aligns with the dying person's wishes. Sometimes it does not. That is where the plan becomes protective. When a family member wants prayer and the dying person does not. When someone wants visitors and the dying person wants rest. When fear shows up as urgency. When families know what their loved one wants, they can act with confidence instead of fear. The death plan is about advocating for the person whose voice will grow quieter.

We also talk about autonomy in care. About medications. About comfort. About pain relief. Some people go into the dying process knowing they want minimal medication. Others are very clear that they want all the comfort available. These preferences matter, and they need to be communicated clearly, especially to family members who may be helping administer medications alongside hospice.

When the plan is complete, I keep a copy in a binder near the client's bed so family members can reference it at any time. If someone wonders what music should be playing or whether touch is welcome or what scent brings comfort, they do not have to guess. The plan becomes a shared roadmap, reducing confusion and conflict in moments that are already heavy.

It is also important to note that a death plan is not written in stone. Just like all end-of-life planning, it can evolve. What someone wants early in the dying process may change as their body changes. Preferences and needs can shift. The plan is a living document, one that adapts alongside the person it is meant to serve.

At its heart, the death plan is where death becomes personal again.

It gives the dying person something real to hold onto. Choice. Agency. Dignity. It gives families a way to help without guessing, to participate without fear, to show love in ways that truly matter.

And later, when families look back, the plan becomes part of the story. They remember the peace in the room. The light. The smell. The way their loved one was cared for. They do not just remember a death. They remember a moment that was intentional and deeply human.

This work grew out of two parts of my life: my work as a death doula and my life as a mother to a child with autism. Learning about my son's sensory system taught me how powerful sensory experiences are, how deeply they shape regulation and safety. One day, listening to a birth doula talk about creating a birth plan, it clicked. If we plan how we come into the world, why would we not plan how we leave it? So, I started creating sensory-friendly death plans. And everything changed.

Families felt less helpless. Clients felt seen. And the dying process itself became gentler. A death plan cannot stop death from happening. But it can change how it happens. It can turn fear into calm, chaos into presence, and a medical event into something sacred.

One of the most memorable death plans I ever helped create belonged to a woman who wanted her death to reflect the way she had lived her life.

She was a die-hard Beatles fan and insisted that when her time came, The Beatles would be playing on repeat. Their music had been the soundtrack of her life, and she wanted it to be the soundtrack of her final hours too.

She also loved coffee. Not casually. Devotedly. She drank it with breakfast, lunch, and dinner, and her plan was very clear: there should always be a pot brewing so the smell of fresh coffee could fill the air around her.

There were only three people allowed in the room during her labor out: her two adult children and her death doula. Me.

She was always cold, the kind of person who lived wrapped in warmth, so she asked to be covered in her favorite soft, fuzzy blankets. She also had one very specific request that made all of us smile. She wanted to leave this world with her hair brushed, her makeup on, and nice, clean clothes. She wanted to look put together.

So her children and I followed her plan carefully.

The Beatles played softly in the background. The smell of coffee drifted through the room. She stayed wrapped in her blankets. And we made sure she looked beautiful. On the day she died, we even remembered to spray her favorite perfume.

She had told us many times that when she died, she believed she would be seeing her husband again for the first time in 10 years. If that was the case, she said, she had to look her best.

Her children took that seriously. It gave them something to do, something loving and purposeful in the midst of a moment that could have otherwise felt helpless. Just a few hours before she died, her daughter carefully touched up her nail polish.

There was so much love in that room that there was barely any space left for fear. It is a moment I will never forget.

Legacy Projects

They say each person dies two deaths: once when their body dies, and again when their name is spoken for the last time. A legacy project is what bridges those two moments. It is a way for someone's love, humor, voice, and spirit to outlive the body that carried it. It becomes something tangible, something intentionally created and left behind, that helps keep a person present in the lives of those who love them.

Legacy work is not about being remembered by the world. It is about being remembered by the people who matter.

Most people hear the word *legacy* and immediately think it has to be something big or impressive. Something creative. Something worthy of being preserved forever. And that assumption stops a lot of people before they ever begin. They will say things like, "I'm not creative" or "I didn't do anything special" or "I don't really have anything to leave."

That could not be further from the truth. Legacy projects look different for everyone. For one person, it might be a collection of recipes written in their own handwriting. For another, it might be a voice recording, a letter, a handmade quilt, or a playlist of favorite songs. Sometimes it is a journal. Sometimes it is a collection of stories. Sometimes it is a single object that carries meaning no one else would ever understand.

And sometimes, it is something incredibly simple.

One time, a legacy project I created for a family was nothing more than a framed piece of paper filled with the phrases their dad used to say. He had all these little quotes he rattled off constantly, the kind that become part of a family's language without anyone realizing it. I started recording them as he said them. After he died, I turned them into a simple document in Canva, printed it, framed it, and gave it to his family.

It was not grand. It was not artistic. It was perfect. Legacy work does not have to be impressive. It has to be personal.

When I am working with clients, legacy projects often grow naturally out of life review. As people reflect on their lives, they almost always talk about what they loved. Gardening. Music. Golf. Poetry. Baking. Writing. Painting. Their children. Their students. Their work. Their values. That is usually when I see the opening.

I will say something like, "You know, that could make a beautiful legacy project."

Sometimes we create them together. Sometimes people want to work on them privately, in their own time, in their own way. Some people find meaning in collaboration. Others find meaning in solitude. What matters is that the project feels aligned with who they are.

One of the most powerful legacy projects I have ever been part of came from a client who was a poet. She had published several books and taught poetry at a university for decades. Words were her life. But after she was diagnosed with terminal cancer during the COVID years, her illness and treatments drained her, physically and creatively. She told me that for years, she had not been able to hear the poems in her head anymore.

About eight months before she died, she and I began working together. One day, in the middle of our conversation, she smiled and said, "Kacie, I can hear my poems again." She said it like someone who had just found a lost part of themselves.

By then, her health had declined too much for her to write. Her hands trembled too much to hold a pen. So instead, she recited her poems aloud to me, and I wrote them down. Every word. Over time, we captured more than 100 poems. Each one was about her adult children, memories of them growing up, her hopes for their futures, and her reflections on motherhood and love. When she felt the collection was complete, we created a book together. She even dictated a note from the author to include at the front.

Her children had no idea we were working on it. After she died, I was able to give each of them a hardcover book filled with their mother's words. Her voice. Her humor. Her wisdom. They held those books like they were holding her.

Legacy work doesn't erase grief, but it gives families something to return to when the absence feels unbearable. Something to hold when they miss the sound of their person's voice or the feeling of their presence. Over time, these items often become anchors in grief. Families revisit them on hard days, anniversaries, and milestones. Their meaning deepens as time passes.

Legacy projects are not just for the people left behind. They matter deeply to the dying person as well.

One of the hardest parts of dying for many people is knowing they will not be there to support their loved ones through the grief of their passing. Creating a legacy project gives them a way to continue caring after death. It offers purpose at a time when so much feels out of control. It gives them something to focus on besides fear. Something that says, "I can still help."

For some people, that looks like letters for future milestones. I once worked with a young mother who was leaving behind a 12-year-old daughter. She created greeting cards for moments she knew she would miss. Graduation. A wedding day. The birth of a first child.

Each card was written with love and intention, meant to be opened when the time came.

For others, legacy work might look like recorded stories, messages for grandchildren, playlists, artwork, or even a scholarship created in their name. I once supported someone who created a scholarship for an art college, honoring her career as an art professor and ensuring her love of creativity would continue to support others.

Legacy work is not limited to objects. It is about transmission. Values. Love. Memory.

Timing matters here. Legacy work is best introduced early, while people still have energy, cognition, and the ability to participate fully. Early on, people can share ideas, make decisions, and contribute meaningfully. When legacy work is delayed too long, opportunities can be lost. Cognition may decline. Energy may fade. What could have been created together may no longer be possible. That said, legacy work is not a deathbed activity. It can happen at any point in life.

Legacy is not something you rush at the end. It is something you live into. I do legacy work regularly myself. I keep a journal for each of my boys, writing notes, messages, and letters to them over time. Someday, long after I am gone, they will be able to read my words and hear my voice across the years.

When I teach doulas about legacy projects, I remind them that there is no one right way to do this work. Some people will dive in eagerly. Others will need gentle invitations. Some will want support. Others will want privacy. The goal is never perfection. It is connection.

Everyone wants to be remembered. Everyone wants to believe they mattered. Legacy projects give people that chance. They keep stories alive. They soften grief. And they leave behind something that says, clearly and lovingly, "I was here."

CHAPTER 9

Active Dying and After-Death Care

The Active Dying Phase

This is the part of death that people fear the most.

This is not because it is violent or chaotic, but because it is unknown. Active dying is rarely talked about honestly, and when it is, the conversation is often wrapped in euphemisms or rushed explanations. That silence leaves families unprepared for what they will see, what they will feel, and what it will be like to sit beside a body that is learning how to let go.

In my work, I don't avoid this phase or soften it with vague language. I name it early, and I talk about it often. By the time a person enters the active dying phase, it is not the first time anyone has heard those words. My families already understand what it means, because it is something we have been walking toward together all along.

I often describe active dying as *the moment when the physical work of living gives way to the spiritual work of leaving*. I also call it what it truly is: a labor out of life. The body is not failing. It is working. It is doing exactly what it was designed to do. Just as it once labored to be born, it now labors to finish the job of living.

People almost always want to know how long this phase lasts. They want a timeline. Something they can hold onto. I usually tell them that active dying often unfolds over about three to fourteen days.

Sometimes it is shorter. Sometimes it stretches longer. And sometimes it does not follow any expectations at all. Bodies do not follow scripts. There is no clock. Each death is its own journey, and no two look the same.

When the body begins this labor, the changes come slowly at first and then with more momentum.

Breathing is usually the first thing families notice. It begins to change in ways that feel unsettling if you are not prepared for it. Breaths may become shallow, then quick, then slow again. There may be long pauses between breaths, followed by several close together. Families often find themselves counting, holding their own breath, waiting anxiously for the next inhale. I gently remind them that this pattern is normal. The body is conserving energy. It is finding a new rhythm as it prepares to rest.

As circulation slows, the hands and feet cool. Skin tone changes. Mottling appears, those marbled patterns of purple and blue that spread as blood moves inward toward the heart and vital organs. The body becomes lighter, drier, more fragile. Lips crack. Eyes glaze.

Breathing often sounds different during this time. Sometimes there is a soft rattling noise with each breath, caused by relaxed muscles and resting fluid in the throat. This is called the *death rattle*. While it can sound alarming to those listening, it is not painful for the person experiencing it. This is a normal part of the bodies labor out.

Most people sleep more and more as this phase deepens. They are still here, but they are no longer anchored in the same way. Communication simplifies. A nod. A squeeze of the hand. A faint smile. Sometimes nothing at all. But hearing is the last sense to go, and I remind families of this often. Your person can still hear you, even when it seems like they can't. Every whisper. Every laugh. Every "I love you." Words carry weight here. They matter more than people realize.

One of the most difficult transitions for families during active dying is watching their loved one stop eating and drinking. This is where fear often takes over. We have been taught our entire lives that food and water are the most basic requirements for survival. And that is true when the body is trying to live. But the body that is actively dying is no longer working toward survival.

As the organs and systems begin to shut down, the body no longer needs fuel. Appetite fades naturally. Thirst diminishes. This is not starvation. This is the body conserving energy and preparing to let go. I encourage families to offer food or fluids only when the person asks for them because forcing intake can cause discomfort.

As digestion slows, food can sit heavily in the stomach and intestines, leading to bloating, nausea, or constipation because the body no longer has the strength to process it. The kidneys are also slowing, losing their ability to filter fluids effectively. Extra fluids can pool in the body, increasing congestion and discomfort. Even with education, this is incredibly hard for families. Love wants to feed. Love wants to fix. But the most compassionate thing you can do is trust that the body knows how to die.

As awareness shifts, other changes often appear. Some people become restless. Some pick at sheets or blankets, their sensory system no longer tolerating the feeling of fabric against their skin. Others may want to remove clothing entirely. We don't always know why this happens. What matters most in these moments is comfort. If someone wants the blankets off, we remove them. If they want the room quiet, we quiet it. And if they want to die naked, then they die naked.

Many people also begin seeing or speaking to people who are not physically present, long lost loved ones. This happens far more often than most realize. They may talk to parents who died years ago, siblings, friends, and my favorite. . .beloved pets who have died in the past. I prepare families for this well before it happens, so they are not frightened or confused. This is not hallucination in the way people imagine. It is part of the transition. It's also a sign that we are getting closer to the end.

People may also begin speaking in symbolic language. They might say things like, "I'm going home now" or "My mom is coming to get me," even if their mother has been dead for decades. These moments are deeply meaningful. They offer a glimpse into where the person's mind and spirit are traveling. I encourage families to lean into these moments rather than shutting them down.

Death is deeply spiritual in ways most people never experience until they are sitting right in the middle of it. During active dying, it often feels as though a person is a little bit here, and a little bit wherever they are going next. Being present for that transition is an honor. It is intimate, humbling, and profound. I tell every one of my clients that I don't know what happens after death. I don't claim to know where they go, or if they will be able to come back and find me. But I always tell them that if they can, they better. And they better leave me signs, so I know they were here. And you better believe I find signs all the time. I truly believe the people I have walked with are still present in some way, guiding me forward just as I once guided them through their leaving.

One of the most beautiful and misunderstood parts of the dying process is something called terminal lucidity. It is what I describe as the body's final spark before the last exhale. A sudden burst of clarity and energy that can look, for a moment, like a miracle.

Someone who has been unresponsive for days may suddenly open their eyes, sit up, crack a joke, ask for their favorite meal, or tell everyone in the room how much they love them. Families who have not been prepared for this often think their person is getting better. They feel hope rush back in, only to be devastated when death follows shortly after.

Terminal lucidity is not recovery. It is a gift.

It is the body offering one final moment of connection before letting go. When families understand this ahead of time, they do not miss it in confusion or false hope. They recognize it for what it is: sacred, fleeting, and profoundly human. I always tell them, if you are one of the lucky ones who gets this moment, don't waste it. Sit close. Hold their hand. Laugh if they laugh. Cry if you need to. Just be there. What follows soon after is death, and this final burst of energy is their soul's way of saying goodbye on their own terms.

Another major fear people carry into death is pain. Many assume that dying is always painful. It isn't. I have seen people die peacefully, without needing a single dose of pain medication at all. For some people, depending on their disease process, pain can be part of the experience. But even then, it is not something they are left to endure alone. Hospice is incredibly skilled at managing comfort in whatever way is needed, adjusting medications and care to meet the body where it is. Sometimes the body is already at peace on its own. Other times, comfort is supported and maintained with intention. Either way, the goal is the same: comfort, dignity, and relief. Dying is not suffering. It is surrender. It is the body exhaling its last bit of effort and the soul slipping quietly into whatever comes next.

Another common misunderstanding is the belief that the dying person is unaware of what is happening around them. I have seen too much to believe that. I have watched breathing steady the moment a loved one takes their hand. I have seen tears roll down cheeks after someone whispered, "It's okay to go." I encourage families to speak love aloud. Say what you need to say, even if you think your person cannot hear it. I promise you, they can.

As the body continues to shut down, more physical signs appear. Urine output decreases and darkens as the kidneys slow. Bowel movements become infrequent, though many people will have one very large (I'm talking *huge*) final bowel movement near the end.

The muscles of the jaw relax, often leaving the mouth open. Facial expression softens and becomes still. Body temperature may fluctuate. Someone may feel warm one moment and cool the next. Fevers can come and go. These are all signs of systems powering down.

Families move through a wide range of emotions during this phase. Anticipatory grief shows up for almost everyone. Grief begins before death arrives. There is fear of missing the moment, fear of leaving the room, fear of doing something wrong. People become exhausted and hypervigilant, afraid to rest. Guilt often creeps in.

I remind families of this often: there is no award for burning yourself out at the bedside.

If you have ever spoken to someone who has had a near-death experience, you'll notice a common theme in their stories. They often describe floating above their body, watching what is happening below. They can see the room. They can see the people. They are aware of the energy and the love surrounding them, even though they are no longer experiencing things in a physical way. I like to believe the active dying phase is similar. That as the body begins to shut down, the person is no longer confined to it in the same way.

Because of that, I tell families this: your person knows you were there. They know who showed up. They feel the love you poured into them, regardless of how long you sat at the bedside. Whether you stayed for hours or stepped out to rest, eat, cry, or simply breathe, it does not erase your presence. Presence is not measured in minutes. It is felt.

Some people choose to die alone. They are private, even at the end. Despite your best efforts, they may wait for the moment when you step out of the room. This does not mean you failed. It means they left exactly how they wanted to. Your presence still mattered, even if you were not there for the final second.

The moment of death itself is often quieter than people expect. Breathing becomes so shallow and sporadic that it can be difficult to recognize the final breath. There are usually long pauses, periods of apnea, sometimes several moments that feel like endings before the true last exhale. And then, there is silence.

The body has finished its labor.

Understanding the dying process is part knowledge and part trust. The more we understand what is happening, the less fear it carries. But not every moment needs explanation. Sometimes the most powerful thing you can do is sit quietly, breathe with them, and witness the body doing what it was always meant to do.

Let go.

When someone enters the active dying phase, everything shifts. Up until this point, the dying person has needed so much from me. We've spent months talking, planning, reflecting, creating legacy projects, laughing, crying, reviewing a whole lifetime. I've helped them feel calm, in control and ready. But when they begin actively laboring out of life, their needs change. Now, they don't need my words or my ideas as much. They just need my presence. In this shift, the family begins to need more support now than they ever did before.

This part is often surprising for new doulas. We are trained helpers. We like to *do*. But active dying asks something different of us. It asks us to be still. To soften. To stop fixing and start witnessing.

This part of the work becomes quieter. It's about being near them, making sure everything unfolds according to their death plan, adjusting small comforts along the way. I might hold their hand if touch soothes them. I might whisper gentle reminders that it's okay to go, that they're safe, that it's time to make the transition we've talked about for so long.

Sometimes that looks like smoothing a sheet, dimming a light, turning off a TV that no longer serves a purpose. Other times it means making sure their music of choice is on and that the surroundings are just as they wanted them. The work becomes subtle. But it matters.

I am always paying attention to the room. The energy. The temperature. The sounds. Active dying is not just happening in the body. It's happening in the space around it. My role is to tend to all of it.

But while the dying person begins to release, the family starts holding tighter. That's where my focus shifts. The energy I once poured into my client now moves to their loved ones. They're the ones sitting at the bedside for hours, sometimes days or weeks, watching every breath, afraid to leave even for a moment. They need someone to hold them steady.

Families are often terrified they will miss something. That they will step away at the wrong moment. That leaving the room means abandoning their person. I gently remind them that love is not measured in minutes or proximity. It's measured in presence, and presence looks different for everyone.

I try to care for the loved ones the same way the dying person would if they were still able to. I show up with bagels and coffee. I remind them to eat. I give them permission to go take a shower, to get some air, to sleep. Sometimes, I just sit beside them so they don't feel alone in the waiting. Grief begins long before the final breath, and my job is to help them survive this tender, exhausting stretch of time.

I also normalize what they're feeling. The irritability. The numbness. The sudden waves of emotion that come out of nowhere. Anticipatory grief can be disorienting, and families often feel guilty for how they're reacting. I remind them that there is no "right" way to sit at a bedside.

By this point, because of all the planning we've done together, most families are surprisingly calm. They're sad, of course, but they understand what's happening because we have been preparing for it. There's minimal chaos, minimal panic. We've usually spent months working together, preparing for what's to come, so now my presence can feel like a continuation, not a rescue.

There are still tears. There's still heartbreak. But when you've built trust and prepared them with honesty, even the grief feels grounded. I make sure I'm grounded, too. I'm calm and steady in the room, always the pillar of support everyone can lean on. And then, when it's over, I cry the whole way home if I need to. That's part of my ritual.

I teach my students that the most important thing at the bedside is to stay human. Be calm, cool, collected, and strong, but don't lose your warmth. This is not the time to perform professionalism. This is the time to be real.

Talk to your client like you always have. They might not answer, but they can hear you. They're still here, in some way.

I also remind doulas that consistency matters. The voice your client has come to trust should not suddenly disappear just because their body is changing. Familiarity brings comfort, even when consciousness shifts.

Keep up the rituals that comforted them in life. Those tiny acts of care tell the soul it's safe to go. They say, "Nothing about you has been forgotten." Ritual does not have to be elaborate to be powerful. It just has to be personal.

I once had a client who adored fresh-cut flowers. Even as she weakened, she made sure there were always blooms by her bed, first by picking them herself and then by having them delivered. When she began actively dying, I showed up every day with new flowers and replaced the wilted ones. I wanted her last days to look and smell just like her living ones.

Another client kept a bottle of holy water by her bedside and sprayed herself every morning. When she couldn't do it anymore, I did it for her. I misted her wrists, her neck, and whispered, "I got you."

These little rituals may seem small, but they're what hold the sacred together. They remind everyone, family, doula, and soul, that dying isn't the end of care. It's the continuation of love, carried right up to the final breath.

Holding Vigil

If the doula's role during active dying is about steady support over time, the bedside vigil is about presence in the moment. It is where everything slows, deepens, and becomes sacred.

The bedside vigil is the most sacred part of this work. It's where everything we've planned, prepared, and taught finally settles into quiet. This is the time when the body is doing the labor of dying, and we, the doulas, hold the space around it.

Vigil is not about action. It's about attention.

Holding vigil isn't one specific act, it's all of it. It's tending to the environment, watching over the dying person, comforting their family, and sensing what the room needs moment by moment. Sometimes it's reading softly from a book they loved. Sometimes it's sitting in absolute silence, just breathing with them. Sometimes it's gentle touch, a cool cloth, Reiki, music, or prayer. The details depend on their death plan, but the energy is always the same, calm, grounded, and full of love.

Vigil is fluid. It shifts from hour to hour, sometimes minute to minute. What felt right in the morning may feel intrusive by evening. A song that once soothed may suddenly feel like too much. A room that felt warm may now need air. The work is staying attuned, not attached.

When I sit bedside, I pay attention to everything. The tone of the room. The family's energy. The rise and fall of the breath. I notice if there's tension, discomfort, or restlessness, and I try to bring ease where I can. A dying body can feel what's around it, so it's my job to make sure the energy is soft. The lights low. The music right. The voices gentle. Everything about the space should feel like peace.

I also pay attention to what doesn't belong anymore. Extra people lingering out of obligation. Conversations that drift toward logistics or conflict. The television left on because no one knows how to turn it off without feeling guilty. Part of holding vigil is protecting the space, gently and respectfully, so it can remain sacred.

One woman I sat vigil with was deeply spiritual and often said she hoped her mother, who had died 10 years earlier, would come for her when it was time. In her final days, she told me she could feel faint tapping on her arm when she was half-asleep, as if someone were trying to get her attention. Then she started seeing what she described as an angel standing in the doorway.

Her family didn't know what to make of it. They were torn between comfort and concern. I reassured them that nothing about this felt frightening or wrong. It felt like anticipation.

On her last day, she seemed to hover between both worlds. I took her hand and called her mother by name. I said, "She's ready. Her body is tired. Her soul is ready. It's time to come get your daughter and walk her home." I felt her hand give mine the softest squeeze, followed by one long, deep sigh, and then she was gone. I'll never know what truly happened in that moment, but I like to think her mother was standing right there, waiting, and that gentle squeeze was her way of saying thank you.

This is what vigil is, the stillness that holds the extraordinary. It's the bridge between life and whatever comes next.

When I train doulas, I remind them not to fear this time. Vigil can feel intimidating at first because it strips away the urge to fix or perform.

The energy in the room often changes as death approaches. You can feel it. The air feels heavier or quieter. Time seems to stretch. Don't be afraid of that shift. Don't rush to fill it. Don't pull people out of it. Let it be. There is nothing to accomplish here. There is only presence. Don't be afraid to speak either. Talk to your client. Call them by name. Say the things that matter. Call in whatever higher energy feels right for them, whether that's ancestors, loved ones, God, the universe, or something unnamed. You're not there to orchestrate anything. You're there to witness the most natural process in the world.

Presence means more than you think. You might not say a word, but your calm becomes everyone's calm. Your steadiness gives the family permission to soften. The dying person can feel that, even if they can't speak it.

At the bedside, less is often more. You don't have to fill the silence. You don't have to create a perfect moment. You don't have to say the right thing. Just be there. Because in that stillness, in the soft hum of breathing and the quiet knowing of goodbye, life gently hands itself back to the universe.

Tips for Holding Vigil

- **Trust the quiet.** Silence is not emptiness; it's medicine. Let it stretch longer than feels comfortable before speaking.
- **Match the room.** If the family is whispering, whisper. If they are reminiscing, smile and join softly. Your energy sets the tone.
- **Tend to the environment.** Lights, sounds, smells, and temperature matter more than people realize. A peaceful space supports a peaceful transition.
- **Keep the body comfortable.** Notice small things: dry lips, twisted sheets, loud machines, and fix what you can. Comfort is care.
- **Hold space, not control.** You can't choreograph a good death. Your job is to tend, not direct. Allow the process to unfold.
- **Stay grounded.** Plant your feet, breathe deeply, and regulate your own nervous system. Families will mirror your steadiness.

- **Don't over-explain.** When physical changes happen, offer reassurance in short, calm sentences: "This is normal. The body knows what to do." Then return to stillness.
- **Use ritual wisely.** Light a candle, play music, pray, or sit in silence. Let the dying person's values guide the moment.
- **Protect the space.** Gently limit interruptions, unnecessary visitors, or distractions that pull attention away from the moment.
- **Exit gently.** If you need to step out, say where you're going and why. Leave your calm behind like a blanket in the room.

After-Death Care

When death finally comes, there's no need to rush. This is often the first moment in days or weeks when time feels like it stops instead of stretches. The waiting is over. The work of the body is complete. What remains is presence.

I often tell families we don't have to rush anything. We can sit for a while. We can breathe. We can cry. We can just be. Some families want to hold their person's hand. Some want to talk. Some want to say prayers or share memories. Some simply sit in silence, stunned by the stillness.

Many families are surprised by how peaceful the room feels after the final breath. Even when the death has been long and hard, there is often a noticeable shift. The tension lifts. The room softens. The work is done.

Every family arrives at this moment differently. Some have been sitting vigil for days, exhausted from the long stretch of waiting. For them, the final breath feels like both release and relief. They're ready for what comes next. Others are startled by the stillness, unsure of what to do, unsure of what happens now.

That's when I gently explain what will unfold once hospice is called. I remind them that when hospice arrives, things will move quickly. The nurse will pronounce the death. Phone calls will be made. The funeral home will be notified. The equipment company will be contacted. Within a few short hours, the bed, the oxygen machine, the medications, the sounds and movement that have filled the house for weeks or months will be gone.

It can feel jarring how fast the world resets itself. One moment the room is full. The next moment is quiet and empty, I always encourage families to take their time before that happens. Stay a little longer. Touch their person's face. Wrap them in a favorite blanket. Brush their hair. Sit in the quiet. This is a once-in-a-lifetime moment, the last time you will ever share this kind of space together.

There is no reason to rush past it.

What happens next depends entirely on the family. Some want to be very involved in caring for the body. Others want to step back and let hospice or the funeral home take the lead. Every response is valid. Every comfort level is different. My role is never to push, only to offer.

After-death care can include many things, or just one simple act:

- Washing the body gently
- Dressing them in favorite clothing or pajamas
- Brushing hair or applying lotion
- Placing meaningful items nearby
- Saying prayers, blessings, or goodbyes
- Sitting quietly and holding their hand

Some families want ritual. Others want privacy. Some want both, at different moments. I meet them exactly where they are and adjust as the moment unfolds.

I worked with a client in her late forties who was dying of MS. She had an 11-year-old daughter who adored makeup. Doing her mom's makeup had become a daily ritual between them, a soft, loving routine that gave them both something beautiful to hold onto.

After her mother died, her daughter asked if she could do her makeup one last time, so she'd look beautiful for the funeral. I gently washed and prepared her mother's body while her daughter applied her favorite lipstick, brushed out her hair, and even gave her a fresh manicure. There was no fear in the room. Only love.

The little girl talked to her mom the entire time, the same way she always had. When she finished, she leaned in close and whispered, "There. Perfect."

That's what after-death care can be: love made visible.

When I teach doulas about this time, I remind them that after-death care is not a checklist. It's a relational moment. It requires patience, sensitivity, and deep respect for the family's emotional state. Some families will want guidance. Others will want space. Some will fall apart. Others will move with surprising steadiness. All of it is normal.

This is also the moment when many families begin to understand something important: the body is no longer their person, but it still deserves care. It is the vessel that carried them through every experience of their life. Treating it gently is one final act of love.

After-death care is not about cleaning up what's left. It's about honoring what remains. It's about tending to the body with the same reverence you would give a sacred altar. Because that is exactly what it is.

Closing the Circle

Every death marks an ending, but for those of us who do this work, it also marks a return. A closing of the circle. We've walked with someone from the very first conversation about their fears to the final exhale, through planning, vigil, and silence. When that journey completes, it's not about leaving. It's about honoring what was shared and allowing it to settle into the part of us that holds all the people we've ever cared for.

My work doesn't stop at the last breath. I always tell families that I'll be there, and I mean it. I attend the funerals of all my clients. For some families, I'm a quiet presence sitting toward the back, offering support without being seen. For others, especially when there isn't much family around, I'm helping plan, organizing, or standing front and center beside them. I fill whatever space they need me to fill. It's never about formality or titles. It's about showing up.

In the days immediately after a death, I stay close. I check in daily at first, a quick text, a phone call, sometimes stopping by in person if it feels right. Those early days can feel disorienting, like the house is suddenly too quiet, like the world moved on without asking permission. Then, as time stretches out, my check-ins become weekly for a while. After that, they're more sporadic. A message to say I'm thinking of them. A photo that reminded me of their person. A simple "How are you today?"

It goes both ways, too. Families will send me pictures or memories out of the blue, reminders that the connection doesn't end with death. We stay in touch long after the services are over. Many of my families follow me on social media, and I follow them. I love watching them slowly return to life, to laughter, to moments of joy that once felt impossible. I always reach out on the anniversary of their person's death. That day never goes unacknowledged.

Some clients even plan ahead for that continued care. They build it right into their end-of-life plan. They'll arrange for me to meet with their loved ones weekly for 12 weeks after their death, creating structure and support during those fragile first months. During those visits, we talk, cry, laugh, and process together. It's part of what I promised their person before they died, that I would help make sure their people make it out of this whole.

When the body has been tended to and the family finally begins to rest, I take a quiet moment alone. I always speak to my clients after they die. Always. I believe that in those first hours and days after they transition, they are still very much around. I talk to them, out loud. I thank them for trusting me to be there through it all. I ask them to keep watching over me, to guide me, to nudge me when I'm wandering off course. And honestly, some of them absolutely do. I can feel it. I thank them for what they taught me, for the reminders they left behind about what it means to be alive.

Each death teaches me something different. One reminds me about love. Another about forgiveness. Another about the grace of letting go. But they all return me to the same truth. This work isn't just about death. It's about connection. It's about witnessing the full spectrum of what it means to be human, the laughter, the fear, the beauty, the surrender. I walk away changed every single time.

When we close the circle with one client, we don't walk away empty. We carry their stories forward. They quietly shape how we show up for the next family, the next bedside, the next moment of stillness. They shape how we move through our own lives, how we love, how we listen, how we pay attention.

That's the sacred rhythm of this work: life, death, reflection, renewal.

And when the room is quiet again and the circle is complete, we turn our attention inward. We begin another kind of tending. The care of ourselves. Because the same hands that hold the dying must also learn to hold their own heart.

PART III

The Doula as Professional

CHAPTER 10

Boundaries, Burnout, and Balance

The Emotional Cost of This Work

There's a cost to doing this sacred work, not in money, but in heart, body, and spirit.

Death work asks something of you long before it ever pays you. It asks you to show up fully present in moments most people spend their lives avoiding. It asks you to sit with fear, uncertainty, grief, anger, regret, and love all tangled together. And then it asks you to go home, make dinner, pick your kids up from school, and pretend you didn't just witness the most intimate moments of someone else's life.

Doing death work is heavy in a lot of ways. You're walking into people's deepest pain, sitting with their fear, holding their grief, and trying not to take it home in your own pocket. Some days, you're watching families say things they'll regret. Other days, you're watching someone suffer because they wouldn't advocate for themselves. And then there's the business side of it, the constant explaining of who we are, what we do, and why this work matters. Being a death doula means living in a perpetual TED Talk.

No one really prepares you for how much emotional labor that last part takes. Educating, translating, justifying your existence in rooms that don't always want to hear it. That effort alone can drain you in ways that have nothing to do with grief.

The emotional cost doesn't hit all at once. It creeps up slowly, like when you've been holding your breath for hours and suddenly realize your chest hurts. For me, it shows up as exhaustion, irritability, tears in the car, the whole shebang. Sometimes it looks like numbness instead. Not sadness. Just. . .flat. I've seen so much death in my life that there are many moments when my system goes quiet inside. That doesn't mean I don't care. It means my nervous system is protecting me.

I don't experience grief the way most people do. When my clients die, I'm not devastated, or even sad at all. I don't feel crushed by heartbreak. Their death is the outcome we were preparing for. I helped them have the best exit possible. And now, in my worldview, they're still around me, just not in a different way than they were before. That clarity is part of why I'm made for this work. If you're wired similarly, that doesn't make you cold. It makes you honest.

When I was a nurse, burnout was worn like a badge of honor. The more hours you worked, the more shifts you picked up, the better nurse you were. Never mind that you were running on caffeine, adrenaline, and spite. Healthcare culture teaches you to burn yourself out and then take a "vacation" to fix it. That is, if you can beg hard enough for any days off. I left that world because I didn't want to spend my life sprinting toward empty.

As doulas, we have to learn a new rhythm. We can't wait until we're falling apart to start caring for ourselves. I tell every new doula this, and I wish someone had drilled it into my head earlier: *self-care isn't what you do when you're burnt out. It's what keeps you from getting there in the first place*. You can't pour from an empty cup, and you can't hold someone's death while you're running on fumes.

These days, self-care isn't a reward. It's on my schedule. I don't chase it when I'm falling apart. I guard it like oxygen. Some days it's a walk in nature. Some days it's silence and coffee. Some days it's saying "nope" to one more email and not explaining myself. I don't apologize for it anymore, because caring for myself is part of the job description.

Death work costs you something, yes, but it also gives something back. It teaches you to live slower, love deeper, and find humor in the chaos. It reminds you that you can hold the heaviest moments of a person's life and still find joy in your own. That balance, the ability to grieve and laugh in the same breath, is what keeps us human in this work.

There's also a strange duality that comes with this work. You can spend an entire day sitting with someone who is dying, holding space for the most vulnerable moments of their life, and then find yourself laughing at something ridiculous on the drive home. That contrast can feel jarring at first. It can even feel wrong. But it isn't. It's your nervous system finding equilibrium. It's your humanity insisting on staying intact.

This work sharpens your awareness of life in ways that are hard to explain to people who don't live this close to death. You notice small things more. Sunlight through a window. A quiet house. The weight of silence after a long day. You also lose patience for nonsense. For urgency that isn't real. For drama that doesn't matter. That shift can be isolating at times, especially when the people around you don't quite understand why you've changed.

I've had to learn how to reintegrate myself into the world after sitting at a bedside, how to re-enter my own life gently, and how to remind myself that while death is always present, it doesn't get to consume everything else I love. That takes practice. It takes awareness. And sometimes it takes messing it up and realizing you've been carrying too much for too long.

There is a quiet discipline to this work that no one talks about. It's the discipline of noticing yourself. Of recognizing when you're becoming short-tempered, detached, or numb. Of catching the signs early instead of pushing through them. Death work doesn't usually break you all at once. It wears you down in small, almost invisible ways if you're not paying attention.

And here's the part that matters most: *none of this means you're doing it wrong.*

Feeling tired doesn't mean you're not cut out for this work.
Feeling numb doesn't mean you've lost your compassion.
Needing distance doesn't mean you care less. It means you are human, doing work that asks you to repeatedly sit in the deepest parts of the human experience.

The people who last in this field aren't the ones who give everything they have until there's nothing left. They're the ones who learn when to hold close and when to step back. They're the ones who understand that being good at this work doesn't mean sacrificing themselves for it.

Death work will always ask something of you. That's unavoidable. But it should never take more than you are willing, able, and resourced to give. Learning that distinction is not selfish. It's essential.

Because if you want to do this work well and if you want to do it for a long time, you have to pay attention to what it costs you. Not with fear. Not with guilt. But with honesty.

That awareness is where sustainability begins.

Boundaries, Burnout, and Balance

One of the hardest lessons in death work is that compassion without boundaries will chew you up and spit you out. Doulas have huge hearts. It's what makes us good at what we do. But that same heart can become our downfall if we're not careful. We want to be everything for everyone: the guide, the fixer, the comforter, the therapist, the family referee, the snack-bringer, the shoulder to cry on. We step in where systems fail. We fill gaps no one else wants to fill. And if we're not intentional, we slowly start giving pieces of ourselves away without realizing it.

Here's the truth no one likes to say out loud: you cannot be all things to all people and remain intact.

Most doulas don't struggle with showing up. We struggle with stepping back. We struggle with saying no. We struggle with trusting that the care we provide is enough, even when we're not available 24/7. Early in my career, I learned that lesson the hard way.

I once said yes to taking on two clients who lived far from each other and whose timelines ended up overlapping. Both entered active dying at the same time. I told myself I could handle it. Nurses do 12-hour shifts all the time, right? What I didn't account for was the emotional toll of being fully present at two separate bedsides, in two different homes, with two families who both needed me deeply. For three straight weeks, I lived on caffeine and adrenaline. I drove back and forth, barely ate, barely slept, cried at stoplights, and told myself it was fine because the work mattered.

And it did matter. Both clients had beautiful deaths. But I was wrecked.

That experience taught me something critical: being good at this work does not mean sacrificing yourself for it. It means knowing your limits and respecting them before your body forces you to.

That's when I started creating what a good friend of mine calls *non-negotiables*. These are the personal rules that keep me grounded no matter how busy life gets. These are the boundaries I do not bend, not for clients, not for work, not for anyone.

- My phone goes on Do Not Disturb between 9 p.m. and 7 a.m. every single day. You can call or text, and I will get back to you when I'm back on the clock.
- I don't take appointments on Mondays. That's my CEO day.
- I don't schedule evening or weekend work unless a client is actively dying.
- I never miss my kids' school events. They spent years watching me miss those moments when I was a nurse. That chapter is closed.

Your non-negotiables will look different, and that's the point. Maybe it's protecting your mornings. Maybe it's one completely unplugged day a week. Maybe it's no social media after dinner. Maybe it's refusing to answer texts that aren't urgent. Whatever they are, you need them. Write them down. Say them out loud. Tell your loved ones. Tell your clients. Boundaries don't just protect your time. They protect your nervous system.

And a non-negotiable works only if you don't negotiate it.

Burnout doesn't always look like tears. Sometimes it's quieter than that. For me, it starts with fog. My brain feels like static on an old television. I'll be mid-email and suddenly forget what I was saying. I'll reread the same sentence three times. That's my warning sign. That's my body saying, "Hey, we need to slow down."

When that happens, I pause. Not because I'm lazy. Not because I'm weak. But because I've learned that pushing through only makes it worse. After a client dies, especially if the work was intense, I give myself space before jumping back in. I treat that pause like medicine, not guilt.

Balance, for me, looks like quiet. I'm an introvert through and through. When the work gets heavy, I disappear into solitude. Coffee in hand. Cats on my lap. Maybe a little online retail therapy. And when the weather's decent, you'll find me on a trail somewhere, talking to the trees like they're old friends.

Balance is not a formula. It's not a checklist. And it doesn't look the same for everyone. I tell my students that you have to find your own version of peace and then protect it like your paycheck depends on it, because it kind of does.

As a business owner, I've also had to draw boundaries inside my own home. I cannot run a company, support families through death, raise kids, keep pets alive, and cook dinner every night like some domestic goddess. Something had to give. For me, that meant delegating. It meant letting go of the belief that I had to carry every responsibility myself. Some things shifted to their father, like helping with school pickups or handling parts of the evening routine. Some things shifted to my kids, too. They learned how to clean bathrooms, help with chores around the house, and even cook simple meals for themselves on occasion. Letting go of the belief that I had to do everything myself to prove my worth was uncomfortable at first. I was the queen of "I'll just do it myself." But balance required me to release that.

There are also emotional boundaries. As doulas, most of us are not licensed therapists or grief counselors. We are not there to fix families, rescue them from their feelings, or carry their grief for them. Our role is to *sit* beside, *not absorb*. To witness, not solve. To hold space, not take it home. Knowing when to refer out, when to bring in additional support, and when to step back is part of ethical practice.

Boundaries, burnout, and balance exist in a cycle. When one slips, the others usually follow. But when they're tended to together, the work becomes sustainable. You stop surviving it. You stop white-knuckling your way through. You start living alongside it.

And that's the goal. Not martyrdom. Not depletion. Not proving how much you can endure.

The goal is to do this work with your whole heart, without losing yourself in the process.

Self-Care in Practice

Self-care doesn't happen by accident. If it isn't planned, it gets pushed aside. Always. And not because you don't care about yourself but because this work is relentless in what it asks of you. That's why I encourage you to start building self-care into your life now, not when you're burned out or hanging by a thread but as a way of protecting yourself before you get there.

We've all been taught self-care backward. We wait until the tank is bone-dry and then try to fill it with a bubble bath and a glass of wine and call it healing. That's not self-care. That's survival mode with better branding. It's slapping a bandage on a system that's already screaming for rest. Real self-care doesn't show up when you're desperate. It shows up quietly, consistently, long before you hit the wall.

Real self-care is boring sometimes. It's repetitive. It's not sexy. It doesn't make for good Instagram content. It's saying no when you could say yes. It's closing your laptop when there's still work you could do. It's choosing sleep over productivity and rest over proving something. And for people who do death work, that can feel deeply uncomfortable at first, because so much of our identity is wrapped up in being the one who shows up, the one who holds it together, the one who can handle more.

Real self-care means putting yourself on your own calendar and treating that time as non-negotiable. I do it unapologetically, and you should too. If it's not written down, it doesn't exist. If it's optional, it will be the first thing sacrificed.

This work will happily take everything you give it. Always. The only way to survive it long-term is to decide ahead of time what belongs to you and protect it fiercely.

Here's how it works for me. My weekends are chaotic. Three kids, one with autism, and a schedule that could qualify as a full-contact sport. By Monday morning, I'm already tired. So Mondays are what I call CEO Mondays. If you look at my calendar, it's completely blocked off. No meetings. No calls. No work. Just me. Every Monday, without fail. I'm the CEO, and the CEO deserves a full day of rest every single week.

That day can look like anything. Sometimes I walk trails with my coffee in hand. Sometimes I get a pedicure. Sometimes I shop for myself or eat lunch with friends. Other Mondays, I don't even change out of my pajamas. I don't "optimize" it. I don't justify it. I don't turn it into another thing I have to do well. The point isn't what I do. The point is that I give myself permission to do it.

And here's the thing I want you to hear clearly: self-care does not have to be productive to be valid. You do not need to earn rest. You do not need to justify it. You do not need to explain why you deserve it.

Rest is not a reward for suffering enough. It is a requirement for continuing. Especially in work that asks you to hold other people's fear, grief, love, and death.

I'm not here to tell you what your self-care should look like. I don't believe in rules like "this counts" or "that doesn't." For one person, rest might mean a nap. For another, it might mean reorganizing a closet because chaos stresses them out. For someone else, it might be movement, lifting heavy weights, or going for a long run. Some people need quiet. Some people need noise. Some people need stillness. Some people need to sweat it out. The key is this: whatever fills your cup, do more of it, and do it on purpose.

Just make sure you're also giving your body what it needs. Good food. Sleep. Water. Movement. Sunlight. Touch. These are not luxuries. These are basic maintenance requirements for a nervous system that does heavy emotional labor for a living. You cannot sit at deathbeds, regulate other people's fear, and absorb that kind of intensity without tending to your body. It's not complicated. It's consistency.

After heavy work, I always find music helps me reset. I'll get in the car, turn something up that hits the soul, and let it wash the energy off me. I journal. Sometimes it's gratitude. Sometimes it's absolute chaos on the page. I don't censor it. I let whatever needs to come out come out. A little grounding. A little stretching. A little quiet. And I can feel myself come back into my body.

That's the part people don't talk about enough. Death work pulls you out of your body if you let it. It pulls you into your head, into vigilance, into holding and watching and waiting. Self-care is how you come home. It's how you remind your nervous system that you are safe, that you are allowed to rest, that you don't have to be on alert all the time.

I'm not the same person I was when I worked in healthcare. Back then, my nervous system lived in fight-or-flight mode. I was frazzled, wired, exhausted, trying to pour from an empty cup at work and then come home and do it all over again. I couldn't rest without guilt. I couldn't slow down without feeling like I was failing someone. Burnout was normalized. Exhaustion was praised. And I internalized all of it.

The difference now is night and day. I know myself. I know my warning signs. I know when the fog is rolling in. I know when my patience gets short, when my body feels heavy, when my mind starts to drift. And I stop before it becomes a problem. I rest before I collapse. I reset without apologizing for it.

The old me couldn't even take a nap without feeling like I'd let someone down. The me I am now can sleep in, drink my coffee slow, and know that rest isn't lazy. It's sacred. It's the reason I can keep showing up fully for my clients, my family, and myself. It's the reason I can stay present instead of resentful.

This is the kind of self-care I want for every death doula. Not the performative, influencer version with perfect lighting and curated rituals. The real, gritty, soul-saving kind. The kind that keeps you steady when the work is heavy. The kind that lets you feel without drowning. The kind that makes this work sustainable, not just survivable.

When I teach my students about self-care, I tell them to treat it like an appointment they cannot cancel. It is not optional. You wouldn't skip a client visit without notice. So don't skip yourself either. Build self-care into your business plan. Build it into your calendar. Build it into your identity as a professional who plans to be here for the long haul.

If you care for yourself the way you care for your clients, you will feel it. Your energy. Your peace. Your presence. Your ability to stay human in the hardest moments. Those are your tools. Protect them like the sacred things they are.

Energy Exchange

There's a kind of connection that happens in this work that's hard to explain to people who've never done it. It's not just emotional. It's energetic. It's the kind of connection you feel in your body before you can put words to it. Every time I sit with a client, it feels like our souls recognize each other, like there's a quiet knowing that passes between us before anything is ever said out loud.

People trust us with things they've never said to anyone else. Not their spouses. Not their children. Not their doctors. They tell us the fears they keep tucked away, the regrets they don't want to burden anyone with, the strange, looping thoughts that show up when you're dying and suddenly everything feels both sacred and painfully ordinary at the same time. There's an intimacy to those conversations that doesn't exist in many other relationships, and it changes you if you let it.

Because of that honesty, a bond forms that runs deep and fast. It's not unusual for clients to want me nearby more than their own family near the end. That can be confusing for loved ones at first, but it makes sense. I'm the one who isn't afraid of death. I'm not trying to cheer them up or pull them back toward life. I'm willing to sit in the truth of where they are. That kind of presence creates a connection most people never experience in their entire lives.

One of my clients had that kind of energy that fills a room the moment she walked into it. She was funny, sharp, warm, the kind of person who could make you laugh even when things were awful. In her last days, she had what I believe was a burst of terminal lucidity. She'd been mostly asleep for several days, quiet and still, and then suddenly she opened her eyes, looked right at me, and said, "You again? You just can't get enough of me, can you?"

Then she swung her legs over the bed, stood up, something she hadn't done in days, and gave me the biggest hug. The air felt charged, like static right before a storm, but in the best way. I could feel the warmth of her energy surrounding us. It was wild and beautiful and heartbreaking all at once. She died peacefully later that night, but that hug still sits in my chest like a little pocket of light. Moments like that don't fade. They imprint.

That's the part people don't talk about enough. Death work isn't just something you do. It's something you feel. And if you don't learn how to work with that energetic exchange, it can knock you sideways.

A lot of doulas struggle here. They feel other people's emotions like waves crashing into them. They leave client visits feeling wrung out, heavy, or disoriented, not because they did anything wrong, but because they absorbed more than they realized. I don't tend to take energy on in that way, but that didn't happen by accident. It's something I've learned to do intentionally.

Before I enter a client's home, I take a deep breath. I plant my feet. I remind myself that I'm the calm in the room, not the sponge. That distinction matters. I'm here to witness, not to carry. If I feel heaviness trying to settle on me, I consciously release it back into the earth. Not in a dramatic way. Just a quiet internal choice to stay grounded.

That's the key. Learning how to stay connected without carrying. It's like standing in the ocean. You can feel the pull of the waves. You can respect their power. But you don't have to let them drag you under.

I tell students that their energy is sacred. Not in a fluffy way. In a practical, survival sense. If you don't protect it, this work will leave you hollow. Protecting your energy isn't something you do only when you're with a client. It's something you practice all the time. It's how you move through the world.

Nature is my reset button. I use it constantly. Sometimes I walk a trail. Sometimes I just stand on my porch and feel the air on my face until my shoulders drop. I touch trees. I listen to birds. I let my body remember that there is a world beyond sick rooms and oxygen concentrators. It's simple, but it works.

This part of the work isn't something you'll find in a manual. It's learned through presence. Through paying attention to how your body feels when you enter a room and how it feels when you leave. Through noticing what lingers and what clears easily. Over time, you'll find your rhythm. You'll learn what grounds you, what drains you, and what brings you back to center.

The important thing to remember is that energy flows both ways. You give some. You receive some. That exchange is what makes this work both exhausting and holy. The goal isn't to shut yourself off. The goal is to stay open without losing yourself.

ENERGY HYGIENE 101 (DOULA EDITION)

You don't have to be a Reiki master or moon-bathe in quartz crystals to protect your energy, though if that's your thing, go for it. This is about awareness and intention, not perfection. Here's what helps:

1. **Ground before you go in.**
   Before walking into a client's home, take one slow, deep breath. Feel your feet on the ground. Remind yourself quietly, *I'm the calm, not the sponge.*
2. **Let it out.**
   When you leave, don't take the energy home with you. Roll the windows down. Blast music. Cry. Sing. Shake it off. Movement and sound clear more than people realize.
3. **Touch something real.**
   Nature doesn't lie. Touch a tree. Stand barefoot in the grass. Look at the sky. It's the fastest way to remember where your energy ends and the world begins.

4. **Protect your inputs.**
   Don't scroll social media right after being with a dying person. Your nervous system doesn't need another wave of noise. Drink water. Eat something. Breathe first.
5. **Reset with intention.**
   Create one ritual that tells your body the workday is done. Wash your hands. Change your clothes. Take off your shoes at the door. Small signals matter.

Because here's the truth. Death work will fill you up and empty you out, sometimes in the same day. Good energy hygiene doesn't make the work lighter, but it makes *you* steadier. And steadiness is what allows you to keep showing up, grounded, human, and able to do this work again tomorrow.

Grief, Guilt, and Letting Go

People always ask me, "Isn't it hard when your clients die?" And my honest answer usually surprises them: no, not really. I don't say that because I'm cold or disconnected. I say it because I see death differently than most people do. I've sat at hundreds of bedsides and felt the shift that happens when someone takes their last breath. The air changes. The room feels lighter, softer, like something has finally settled. Whatever comes next, and none of us truly know, I've never once felt it was anything bad. It always feels like peace.

By the time my clients die, we've spent months preparing for that moment. We've talked about it openly. We've planned it intentionally. Sometimes we've even laughed about it. So, when it finally happens, it doesn't feel like an ending to me. It feels like completion. Like we did it. All those conversations, all that preparation, every hard moment along the way, it led right here. My heart doesn't break. It swells. I feel gratitude. I feel pride. I feel honored that I got to help someone have the death they wanted.

That doesn't mean I don't care deeply. It means I care honestly. This work isn't about clinging. It's about guiding. And when the journey reaches its natural conclusion, there's a sense of rightness to it. Death, when it's prepared for and supported, doesn't feel violent or wrong. It feels like the final step of something that's been unfolding all along.

I know people hate the phrase "in a better place," but honestly, I believe that they are. By the time a person dies, their body has often been on a slow decline for days, weeks, or months. It can no longer sustain life. So, wherever they're going after this, it has to be better than what their body was doing here. I believe energy never dies. It just changes form. And if that's true, then none of this is truly goodbye.

I also know that not everyone shares that belief, and that's okay. You don't have to know exactly what happens after death to feel at peace with it. You don't have to believe what I believe to move through grief with honesty and self-compassion. All you need is a willingness to let death be what it is, a transition, not a failure.

I always remind students and families that just because *I* experience grief with clarity and calm does not mean that's how everyone else will. Grief is not a performance, and it's not a measure of how much you loved someone. It's simply the body and heart trying to adjust to an absence.

For some people, grief is loud. It comes in waves of sobbing, anger, disbelief, and longing. For others, it's quiet and sneaky. It shows up weeks later as exhaustion, irritability, brain fog, or a sudden ache that seems to come out of nowhere. Some people feel everything all at once. Others feel almost nothing at first and then worry something is wrong with them. Nothing is wrong. Grief has its own timing.

One of the hardest parts of grief is the urge to "do it right." People worry they're grieving too much or not enough. Too soon or too late. Too visibly or too privately. I want to say this clearly: there is no correct way to grieve. There is only *your* way. And that way will change over time.

Letting go doesn't mean forgetting. It doesn't mean moving on or closing a door. Letting go simply means loosening your grip on the moment of loss so you can keep living. It means learning how to carry someone with you without being crushed by their absence. That takes time. It takes patience. And it takes kindness toward yourself.

I often tell families that grief needs movement. It doesn't want to be trapped inside our bodies. Talk about your person. Say their name. Tell their stories. Cry when it comes up. Laugh when something reminds you of them. Write letters. Sit in silence. Walk outside. Feel your feelings. Grief moves best when you let it breathe.

And just as important, give yourself permission to step away from it sometimes. You do not have to sit in your grief constantly to honor it. Distraction is not denial. Joy is not betrayal. Laughing does not mean you are loved any less. Your nervous system needs breaks, especially in the early days.

If guilt shows up, and it often does, meet it gently. Guilt for surviving. Guilt for resting. Guilt for feeling relief after a long illness. Guilt for moments of peace. These feelings are common, but they are not truth. They are the mind trying to make sense of loss. You do not need to punish yourself to prove your love.

For those who feel stuck in the moment of death, who worry about forgetting or moving forward, ritual can help. Light a candle. Create a small space of remembrance. Talk to them out loud. Write things down. Relationships do not end at death. It simply changes form.

I once had a medium tell me that every soul I've ever helped cross over is still with me. That they're all here, guiding me, nudging me in the right direction, protecting me from the dumb decisions I'd probably make on my own. I choose to believe that, because honestly, how else would I have gotten this far? So when things happen in my life or my work, I'll sometimes think, *Was that Lisa helping me? Was that Heidi? Was that Margaret giving me a little push? Did that genius idea just come from Annette?*

Because of that, I talk to them all the time. I thank them when good things happen. I tell them when I'm proud of myself. Sometimes I'll smell a familiar perfume out of nowhere or hear a song that feels like a wink from someone I've lost. It's comforting. I don't see my clients as gone. They're just somewhere else, doing whatever comes next, but still very much part of my life.

What surprises people even more than my lack of sadness is the absence of guilt. I don't feel guilty for not being devastated. I don't feel guilty for laughing after a death. I don't feel guilty for returning to my life. I see grief differently than most people, and that's likely why I'm made for this work.

I also don't carry my clients' deaths the way people expect me to. I don't bottle them up or stack them inside my body. I've learned how to let things move through me instead of lodging themselves deep inside. When I'm tired, I rest. When my energy feels drained, I go outside and let nature recharge me. I laugh a lot, because humor heals just as much as tears do. Sometimes more.

When I teach students, I tell them that grief isn't something to fear or fix. It's not a problem to solve. It's an experience to move through. If you try to outrun it or suppress it, it will find other ways to surface. But if you let it flow, acknowledge it when it comes, and release it when it passes, it doesn't have to consume you.

Some days will feel heavy. The silence will hit harder than expected. Other days you'll feel light, grounded, even grateful to have witnessed something sacred. Both are normal. Both are allowed. There is no single right way to carry this work or this loss.

Death doesn't make me sad. Ignorance of it does. Avoiding it. Denying it. Pretending it isn't coming. That's where the real suffering lives. But when we face death head-on, when we talk about it openly, plan for it intentionally, laugh and cry through it together, we take our power back.

When people ask me if this job ever gets easier, I tell them it's not supposed to. It just gets more meaningful. Every client teaches me something different. And every time I help someone die, a little piece of me comes back more alive.

CHAPTER 11

Working with Hospice and Healthcare Teams

Death Doulas Are Not Hospice

One of the biggest misconceptions people have about death doulas is that we are basically hospice in different clothes. We are not. I understand the confusion. Hospice and death doulas often enter the picture around the same time. We both talk about comfort. We both care deeply about dignity. We both show up when life is narrowing and families are trying to make sense of what is happening. From the outside, it can all blur together.

But the difference is actually simple.

Hospice is **medical end-of-life care**. Death doulas are **nonmedical end-of-life support**.

Hospice teams are made up of nurses, physicians, aides, social workers, chaplains, and bereavement staff. Their role is to manage the clinical aspects of dying. They assess symptoms, order equipment, adjust medications, support comfort, and help families understand what is happening physically. Hospice is built to support the body through the dying process. And when hospice is good, it can be one of the most compassionate and valuable services a family will ever receive.

Death doulas do something different.

- We do not give medications.
- We do not assess symptoms.
- We do not make clinical recommendations.
- We do not override the care plan.
- We are not there to play nurse without a license.

That is not our lane.

Our role is to support the emotional, spiritual, practical, logistical, and human experience of dying.

- We help families understand what is happening in a way that actually lands.
- We sit in the quiet no one else has time for.
- We help families make sense of what is happening when fear and grief make everything feel confusing.
- We help people prepare.
- We help them breathe.
- We help them make meaning.
- We help them feel less alone.

In many ways, we become the project manager of the most important project of all: someone's final chapter.

Hospice and death doulas are not competing roles. They are different roles. And that difference is exactly the point.

I have never seen a family say, "Wow, we had too much support." What I have seen are families drowning between visits, panicking over normal changes, misunderstanding what the nurse said, feeling too terrified to call for help, and carrying emotional weight that no one has had the time to sit with. That is often where the doula enters. Not to replace hospice. Not to compete with healthcare. But to support the parts of dying that medicine, by design, cannot always fully hold.

That is not a criticism of hospice or healthcare. It is simply the truth of the system. Modern healthcare was not designed to hold the full emotional, relational, and spiritual weight of dying. Healthcare teams are working inside time limits, staffing shortages, documentation requirements, and impossible expectations. Even the most compassionate nurse cannot be in five homes at once. Even the best hospice team cannot physically sit at every bedside all day. Families often do not need more credentials in the room. They need more steadiness. More clarity. More human support.

When I explain it to families, I usually keep it simple. **Hospice supports the clinical side of dying. Death doulas support the human side of it.** When you work with both, you get full, well-rounded support.

And when end-of-life care is truly intentional, that is what it should feel like. Not fragmented. Not rushed. Not like everyone is speaking a different language. Intentional care means the body is supported, the family is supported, and the human experience of dying is not treated like an afterthought.

What Collaboration Actually Looks Like

People love to talk about collaboration like it's some lofty professional ideal, a buzzword for conference panels and networking events. But at the bedside, collaboration is much simpler than that. It is not about titles or hierarchy. It is not about being formally recognized. It is not about proving your value with a speech and a laminated brochure. Collaboration, in real life, looks more like: does your presence offer stability or disruption? Healthcare professionals are walking into emotionally loaded environments all day long. They are managing pain, symptoms, family questions, medication changes, charting, supply needs, and a hundred tiny decisions that all matter. They do not need another person in the room making things more confusing. They do not need someone creeping into medical territory. They do not need someone who thinks "support" means giving opinions about medications they do not understand.

When a doula enters the picture, especially in the beginning, the team is naturally assessing. Not judging. Assessing. Who is this person? Do they understand their role? Are they going to calm this room down or light it on fire?

The best way to answer those questions is not with a long explanation. It is with how you show up.

Good collaboration starts with role clarity. I know exactly what belongs to the medical team and what belongs to me. My role is to help families absorb and understand what is happening. Sometimes that means sitting with them after the nurse leaves and helping them make sense of what they just heard. Fear and exhaustion make it hard for people to take in information clearly. So I help slow things down. I help them understand what matters right now, what is normal, and when it is time to call hospice. I am not replacing the nurse. I am reinforcing the care plan in a way the family can actually hold onto.

That builds trust faster than almost anything else.

But collaboration is not only about what you avoid. It is also about what you bring.

I bring steadiness. I bring regulation. I bring language families can understand when fear has scrambled everything they just heard. I help people separate panic from urgency. I remind them to eat, breathe, rest, call hospice when needed, and stop Googling themselves into a fresh emotional crisis. I help the room come down from the ledge.

One hospice nurse once said to me, "I don't know exactly what you do, but whatever it is, the family is always calmer when you're here."

That is collaboration.

Not because I needed her validation to know my role mattered. But because she felt the difference. The family felt the difference. The room felt different.

I remember supporting one family whose loved one was actively dying. The hospice nurse was excellent. She was skilled, attentive, and compassionate. But the family was unraveling. Every change in breathing sent them into panic. Every sound felt like an emergency. They were exhausted, overwhelmed, and terrified they were doing something wrong.

I sat with them. I grounded them. I reminded them what was normal. I encouraged one of them to go eat something. I got another to step outside for air. I slowed the whole emotional temperature of the room down.

When the nurse returned, she did not walk back into chaos. She walked into a steadier room.

Later she pulled me aside and said, "Whatever you did in there made my job easier."

That is the goal. Good collaboration reduces chaos. It does not add to it.

This is also why I do not believe collaboration means shrinking yourself or trying to be invisible. It means being clear. It means being grounded enough in your role that you do not need to perform it loudly. You do not need to compete with medical authority to be valuable. You do not need to over-explain yourself to belong. If you are helping the family feel safer, helping the room feel more regulated, and helping the care team work without extra emotional fallout, then you are already doing the job well.

The best collaboration often looks almost boring from the outside. No drama. No power struggle. No doula trying to be the main character. Just clear roles, mutual respect, and one shared goal: helping a person die with as much comfort, dignity, and support as possible.

Helping Families Understand and Choose Hospice

One of the most important things a death doula can do is help families understand what hospice actually is. Most of the time, I begin working with clients before hospice enters the picture, which means I get to help them understand what hospice is and what hospice is not.

Because let's be honest, the word *hospice* still scares the heck out of people.

For a lot of families, hospice sounds like the official end of hope and surrender to death. It is often introduced in rushed medical conversations, with bad timing, bad phrasing, and all the warmth of a printer manual. Families hear the word and immediately tense up. Someone starts crying. Someone else gets angry. Someone asks how long the person has left, even though no one can answer that with certainty.

So before families can choose hospice well, they usually need someone to help untangle what hospice is not.

Hospice is not giving up. Hospice is leaning in.

It is choosing comfort. It is choosing support. It is choosing a care model that stops asking, “What else can we do to fight this?” and starts asking, “What will help this person live as comfortably and meaningfully as possible now?”

People often think they should wait until the last days of life to bring hospice in, but that does a disservice to both the dying individual and the family. Hospice can offer support in many ways for months before death, and waiting until the very end is rarely the best approach. I tell families all the time, if the doctor has already given you the hospice referral, now is the time. You cannot bring hospice in too early. You can only bring them in too late.

There is this idea that hospice is for the final 24 hours, when everyone is already drowning and half the family is in denial and nobody knows where the morphine is. That is not how hospice works best. Hospice works best when it has time to do what it is actually meant to do: build rapport, educate the family, manage symptoms well, and put supports in place before the crisis hits.

Hospice can provide oxygen, a hospital bed, medications, supplies, symptom management, education, nursing support, aide visits, social work, chaplaincy, and 24-hour access to on-call help. That is huge. Families often do not realize how much support is available until they are already exhausted and wishing they had said yes sooner.

That said, not all hospice companies are created equal.

A doctor’s referral is not a gold star. It does not automatically mean that the hospice your doctor recommended is the best fit, the most responsive, or the most aligned with your family’s needs. Sometimes referrals are based on convenience, habit, contracts, or existing systems, not necessarily quality. In most areas, families are allowed to choose. They are allowed to ask questions. They are allowed to interview more than one hospice company.

I encourage families to interview at least three hospice companies whenever possible, especially if they have the emotional bandwidth to do so. They are not ordering a side salad. This is end-of-life care. The fit matters.

Sometimes I sit with families through their hospice interviews when they want the added support. Whether I am there with them or not, I always arm them with **these five questions**:

1. **What does continuity of care look like?**
   Will the same nurse and aides be coming consistently, or should the family expect a rotating cast of strangers? Continuity matters when you are trying to build trust with the people who will be caring for your loved one.
2. **How quickly can medications and equipment be delivered, especially after hours, weekends, or holidays?**
   Declines do not care that it is Saturday night or Christmas Eve.
3. **How fast can on-call staff get to the home when needed, especially during off hours?**
   Vague answers here are not comforting. You want to know the team will be responsive no matter the time, day, or holiday.
4. **What additional services do you offer?**
   If this matters to your family, ask. Some hospices offer additional services that may help you decide which team feels like the best fit.
5. **What does bedside support look like during the active dying phase?**
   If support does not increase when dying intensifies, families deserve to know that upfront.

I help families pay attention not just to the answers but to the energy. Other questions to consider:

- Are they warm? Clear? Organized?
- Do they speak to the family like human beings or like they are processing a transaction?

- Do they welcome questions?
- Do they seem comfortable with a death doula being involved?
- Do they explain things in a way that feels grounded and compassionate?

I always tell families to pay attention to the vibes. If you interview more than one hospice company, you will usually get a noticeably better feeling from one of them. That matters. This is not the time to talk yourself out of your instincts.

I once worked with a woman who was terminal with cancer and wanted absolutely nothing to do with hospice. She distrusted the medical system deeply and was convinced hospice would take over, force medications, and strip her of control. Meanwhile, she was getting more short of breath by the day. She desperately needed oxygen, but in her mind, accepting hospice meant surrendering her autonomy.

I worked with her for many months. I did not push. I educated.

Gently. Repeatedly. Clearly.

I explained that hospice follows the patient's wishes. I explained that medications are offered, not forced. I explained that accepting support did not mean giving up control. I told her over and over that they could get her oxygen without turning her death into something she did not want.

Eventually, she agreed to interview a few hospice companies and chose to work with one hospice team I trusted.

During the assessment, the nurse checked her oxygen levels and they were dangerously low. Within two hours of signing on to hospice, oxygen was delivered to her home. The relief was immediate. Her breathing eased. Her fear softened. She was shocked by how kind and respectful the team was. She ended up dying peacefully at home weeks later using oxygen only, no medications, exactly the way she wanted.

Hospice did not take over her death. They supported her body.

I supported her emotionally.

That is what good collaboration looks like.

Supporting Families with Hospice, Not Against Them

Even after hospice is involved, families still need a lot of support around understanding how to use it. They often hesitate to call because they do not want to bother anyone. They do not know what counts as urgent. They worry they are overreacting. They second-guess themselves constantly. One of the most common things I do as a doula is remind families that hospice is there to be used. They are not annoying anyone by calling for help. That is exactly what hospice is there for.

Sometimes my role is as simple as saying, "Have you told the hospice nurse about how you're feeling? Why don't you give her a call?"

Sometimes it is the loved ones who need that gentle guidance. As someone moves deeper into their labor out of life, family members are often the ones giving medications and monitoring comfort around the clock. I check in with my clients daily during the active dying phase, and sometimes I can see signs of discomfort even when the person is no longer able to verbalize it. In those moments, family members may need a little help recognizing what they are seeing and knowing it is time to call hospice for guidance on how to keep their loved one more comfortable.

Something important that many families do not realize about hospice is that you are not locked into one hospice company. If you live in an area with several providers, you have the ability to choose the hospice team that feels like the best fit for you and your loved one. And that choice does not disappear after enrollment. If the hospice you initially select is not meeting your needs, you are allowed to switch to a different provider.

Part of the confusion comes from how little education most people receive about hospice in general. Because the word itself carries so much fear, many people picture hospice as a physical place where someone goes to die. In reality, hospice is most often a service that comes to you. The team supports the patient and family wherever they call home. Some communities do have inpatient hospice facilities, but those are typically reserved for situations where symptoms require a higher level of medical management.

Hospice teams do incredibly important work. They guide the clinical side of end-of-life care and help ensure that a person is as comfortable as possible. Many hospice teams provide extraordinary care and compassion during one of the hardest times a family will ever face. At the same time, like any healthcare service, experiences can vary depending on staffing levels, resources, and organizational structure.

Because of that, I always remind families that it is okay to advocate for the level of care their loved one deserves. If the hospice provider they chose is not responding well, communicating clearly, or supporting the family in the way they hoped, they are allowed to explore other options. Switching hospice providers is not uncommon, and it can sometimes make a meaningful difference in the experience of those final months or weeks.

I always say: YODO. You only die once. Your final chapter deserves thoughtful, compassionate care.

Intentional end-of-life care does not happen by accident. It happens when the right support is in place, when families understand their options, and when everyone involved is clear about the role they are there to play. Hospice and healthcare teams carry the clinical side of dying. Death doulas help carry the human side. When those roles work together with clarity and respect, the labor out of life becomes less chaotic, less frightening, and far more supported for everyone involved.

And that matters not only for the families we serve, but for the doulas reading this book and wondering where they fit. This work does not happen in isolation. It happens in relationship. It happens in conversation. It happens in homes, at bedsides, in the spaces between nurse visits, and in the tender moments where someone needs help making sense of what is unfolding. Learning how to work well with hospice and healthcare teams is not separate from being a death doula. It is part of becoming one.

The Larger Healthcare Landscape

Hospice is often the team people associate most closely with the end of life, but it is rarely the only healthcare system involved.

By the time someone reaches the final chapter of life, they may have spent months or years navigating a complex medical landscape. Oncologists, cardiologists, surgeons, hospitalists, primary-care physicians, and palliative care specialists may all have been part of the journey.

Each of these professionals brings important expertise. They diagnose illness, manage treatments, and work to relieve suffering. But healthcare systems are largely built around treatment and intervention. They move quickly. They focus on measurable outcomes. They operate under enormous pressure.

Families, meanwhile, are trying to absorb life-altering information while living through one of the most emotionally overwhelming experiences of their lives.

This is where gaps naturally appear. Not because healthcare professionals lack compassion but because the system itself was never designed to hold the full emotional and relational weight of dying.

Palliative care teams often come closest to bridging that gap. Palliative care focuses on comfort, quality of life, and helping patients navigate serious illness even while treatment is still ongoing. It is not limited to the final days or even the final months of life. Patients can receive palliative care alongside curative or life-prolonging treatments, sometimes for years. When palliative care is involved early, it can dramatically improve the experience for both patients and families.

This is where confusion often happens. Hospice and palliative care are frequently used interchangeably, but they are not the same. Hospice care is designed for those nearing the end of life, typically when curative treatment is no longer being pursued and a physician estimates a limited prognosis of six months or less to live. Palliative care, on the other hand, can begin much earlier in the disease process and does not require a patient to be dying. Understanding this distinction matters, because many people often miss out on the supportive care of palliative simply because they think it is “too soon” for them to get involved or that they are only for the very end of life.

When death doulas and palliative care teams work alongside one another, the support around a patient can become incredibly powerful. The medical team manages symptoms, medications and treatment decisions. The doula supports the emotional, relational, and human experience of what it means to live through a serious illness. The result is care that feels more complete and far less isolating for families.

These collaborations are still evolving. Many healthcare professionals are only beginning to learn about death doulas. Some are curious. Some are cautious. Some have never encountered one before.

But the conversation is growing.

The Future of Collaboration

End-of-life care is slowly changing.

For decades, death has been treated almost entirely as a medical event. But dying is not only clinical. It is emotional, relational, spiritual, and deeply human.

More healthcare professionals are beginning to recognize that excellent end-of-life care requires more than symptom management alone. Interdisciplinary teams already include social workers, chaplains, nurses, and others who provide critical emotional, psychosocial, and spiritual support. And still, even with these roles in place, there are gaps.

Because it is not a lack of skill or compassion. It is often a lack of time, capacity, and continuity.

Patients and families need communication. Preparation. Support. Guidance. They need someone who can stay, who can return, who can walk alongside them through the unfolding of it all.

This is where death doulas naturally fit.

We are not here to replace healthcare professionals. We are here to extend and complement the work they are already doing, helping to ensure that no part of the human experience of dying is left unsupported.

In the years ahead, we will likely see deeper collaboration between healthcare teams, palliative care providers, hospice professionals, and death doulas. When each role is understood and respected, the entire experience of dying becomes more supported for patients and families.

That is the direction this field is moving. And the doulas entering this work will be part of shaping that future.

Because when the right people come together, each holding their piece of the work with care, the labor out of life becomes far less frightening and far more human for everyone involved.

CHAPTER 12

Becoming a Death Doula and Building a Practice

So You Want to Become a Death Doula

At some point, whenever I talk about this work, the same question eventually comes up.

"How do you actually become a death doula?"

It's a fair question, and the answer surprises a lot of people. There is no single official path into this work. No governing body overseeing the field. No universal certification that suddenly declares someone fully prepared to guide others through the end of life. Death doula work is still an emerging profession, which means the landscape is wide open in both beautiful and sometimes confusing ways.

People come to this work from everywhere. Nurses. Social workers. Caregivers. Therapists. Volunteers. People who have spent years around death, and people who simply felt a pull toward it long before they had the language for what that pull meant. But just because there is no official gatekeeper does not mean education doesn't matter.

It matters deeply.

Death work asks a lot of you. You are stepping into people's lives during one of their most vulnerable chapters. Families are scared. Emotions are high. Decisions carry weight. The role of a death doula is not just to care deeply. It is to show up with knowledge, steadiness, communication skills, and a clear understanding of where your role begins and ends.

A good heart is important. Preparation is essential.

That belief is one of the reasons I created Death Doula School. I saw how many people felt called to this work but had no idea where to start, and I also saw how inconsistent the available training could be. Because this field is relatively new, there is no governing body that officially certifies death doulas.

That means when a program offers "certification," what they are really offering is proof that you completed their course. It is not a license and doesn't make one doula more legitimate than another. This is where things can get confusing. Some programs market their certification in a way that makes it seem official or required. Others teach only a small piece of the work, leaving doulas unprepared for the reality of what the role really asks of them. Doulas don't need a fancy title; what they really need is good foundational education. Training that talks about the emotional side of death, but also the practical realities. Training that prepares you for real families, real dynamics, real uncertainty. Training that doesn't romanticize the work, but respects the depth of it.

Because becoming a death doula is not about collecting a title. It's about becoming someone who can walk beside people with steadiness, humility, and skill during one of the most important transitions of their life.

And before anyone ever builds a doula business, finds clients, or prints their first business card, there's a deeper question that matters even more than *how* you become a death doula.

Why? Why this work? Why does it pull on you? Why does it matter to you?

Because long before you build a practice, your "why" is the thing that will anchor you in the moments when the work becomes heavy, complicated, or emotionally intense.

And that's where we're going to begin.

Finding Your Role and Your "Why"

There's a moment in most people's lives when the path stops whispering and starts yelling. Not gently. Not politely. Just loud enough that you can't pretend you didn't hear it.

For me, that moment was COVID.

Before that, I had already been "the death girl" in nursing. I didn't have the title or the language for it yet, but everyone around me knew. I was the one sent into the room when someone was actively dying. The one families clung to because I somehow knew what to say, when to speak, and when to shut up. I wasn't trying to specialize. I wasn't branding anything. I was just. . .good at death. Naturally. Without effort. Without fear.

I didn't realize that was a skill. I just thought it was a weird personality quirk.

Then COVID hit, and everything cracked wide open.

I watched people die fast, scared, and alone. I watched families barred from rooms, final goodbyes reduced to FaceTime screens and muffled voices behind masks. I watched healthcare systems choose efficiency over humanity again and again. And I was standing there, torn between charting, alarms, phone calls, policies, and a human being actively laboring out of life with no one there to witness it.

And without even thinking about it, I kept choosing people over paperwork.

Every single time.

That's when it hit me, not like a gentle realization but like a brick to the soul. I am not built for a version of healthcare where humanity gets sacrificed to documentation. I am built for the threshold moments. The liminal space. The presence part. The part that can't be charted or measured or justified in productivity metrics.

I didn't burn out of nursing. I outgrew it.

So I left. I became a death doula. And I have never once looked back.

People ask me all the time why I became a death doula, and my answer never changes. I didn't choose this. It was written on my soul. I know that sounds dramatic, but it's the only honest answer I have. When you finally step into work you were created for, it doesn't feel like a career decision. It feels like remembering something you already knew.

And then my grandma, my person, became my first true client. When Alzheimer's began taking her, I uprooted my entire life and moved states to be there. I wasn't acting as a nurse. I was acting as an advocate, a guide, a translator, and an emotional anchor. I supported my grandfather, my mom, my uncle with autism, all of us navigating a long, complicated goodbye with no roadmap.

That experience changed me permanently. After she died, something in me settled. It was like a deep internal click that said, this is it. This is what you're here to do.

People love to assume death doulas all look and act a certain way. Soft-spoken. Quiet. Serene. Maybe a little ethereal. I don't buy that for a second. There is no blueprint for a death doula. You don't need a specific aesthetic, personality type, or spiritual alignment. You don't have to talk in whispers or wear linen or say things like "journey" every five minutes.

You just have to feel the pull, the calling.

If you're reading this book, don't overthink it. You probably feel it. That's the qualification. The knowing. The sense that you don't fully understand why you're here, but you know you're supposed to be.

I hear people say all the time, "I don't think I could do this. I'm too empathetic." And that always makes smile. Because that's exactly what makes you good at this work.

Deep empathy isn't a liability in deathwork. It's a compass. When you can truly imagine yourself in someone else's experience, you show up differently. You don't rush. You don't fix. You don't avoid. You stay. Death work requires that kind of heart, paired with the ability to stay grounded inside it.

When I think about who I am as a doula, I'm an advocate, an educator, a steady presence. But I'm also the person who will sit with you in the deepest truth of your life and still make you laugh. I tell my clients all the time, "We're in your final chapter. You know what that means? YODO. You only die once. And we're only accepting the best from here on out."

Humor matters. Joy matters. Dying people deserve both.

My strengths show up without effort. I bring calm where others bring fear. I don't shove death into a dark corner of my mind. I walk right next to it. Death is not my enemy. She's my co-worker. My girl. She's not here to hurt people. She's here to do a job. And I'm here to prepare people for her arrival.

That's my superpower.

However, I didn't start out confident in every area. Money was a big one. There's this unspoken belief that helping someone die should be free, or at least deeply discounted. So, I used to talk about my pricing like I was apologizing for existing. Like feeding my kids was a moral failing.

Almost every client I've ever worked with has said some version of, "How does anyone do this without you?"

The work you offer is invaluable, whether you feel confident yet or not.

If you're looking for signs that this work is calling you, they often sound like this:

- You've always been the one people turn to in crisis.
- Death doesn't scare you the way it scares others.
- You're more comfortable sitting in silence than filling it.
- You feel drawn to end-of-life stories, not repelled by them.
- You can hold heavy conversations without needing to fix them.

That pull matters. Trust it.

And as you move through the rest of this chapter, I want you to carry this one truth with you:

> **Your "why" is the anchor that keeps you from losing yourself in everyone else's chaos.**
>
> **And trust me, there will be chaos.**

Building Trust with Your Community

When I first started as a doula, I thought building trust in my community meant printing a stack of business cards, walking into every hospice and nursing home within a 10-mile radius, and chirping, "Hi! I'm a death doula!" like a deranged Girl Scout selling grief cookies.

And listen. Bless my heart. I tried. I truly did.

What I didn't realize at the time was that trust doesn't come from announcing yourself. It comes from being *known*. And those are very different things.

Trust is not built by showing up once, handing someone a card, and hoping they remember you when their world falls apart three years later. Trust is built slowly, over time, through repeated exposure, shared experiences, and consistency. This is true especially in death work, where people are not just choosing a service. They are choosing a human being to walk them through one of the most vulnerable moments of their life.

That's why networking is wildly underrated in this field.

Not fake networking.
Not "I emailed a funeral home once so I think I'm networking."
I'm talking about actual, grown-up, sometimes uncomfortable networking.

Getting out into your community. Going to meetings. Sitting in rooms with people you don't know. Scheduling one-on-one coffees. Having conversations that aren't about selling yourself but about letting people actually meet you. Not the polished doula version. The real you. The grounded, compassionate, slightly hilarious human they will one day trust with their people.

Because here's the part nobody tells new doulas:

> *Everyone you meet is either going to refer a client to you someday or become a client themselves.*

Everybody dies.
Even professionals.
Even the hospice liaison who seems unfazed by everything.
Even the funeral director who's seen it all.

Sometimes it's the woman you sat next to at a women's networking breakfast. Sometimes it's the colleague you grabbed coffee with for years. Sometimes it's the person who watched you show up consistently in the community and quietly clocked your integrity. And one day, they call and say, "It's my time. I want you to walk me through it."

That's the power of networking.
It widens your world before you even know you need it to.

It leads to speaking at community events.
Getting invited to expos.
Partnering with local organizations.
Meeting professionals who collaborate instead of compete.
Being talked about in rooms you've never even stepped foot in.

If I could tell new doulas one thing about building trust in their community, it would be this:

> **Networking will change your life.**

It changed mine because another doula nudged me into it when I didn't think it mattered. Connections turned into clients. Collaborations. Opportunities. Friendships. Media features. A life I couldn't have planned if I tried.

Your community cannot trust you if they do not know you exist.

So be loud.
Be visible.
Be proud of your work.

And trust will follow.

And if you want to be found locally, here is the most practical advice I will ever give you in this chapter: **make a Google business listing.**

If you are not on Google, you basically do not exist. People need to be able to search "death doula near me" and find you. Don't skip this step. It is not optional.

You Are Your Brand

But here's the deeper truth underneath all that visibility:

You are your brand. Not your website. Not your business cards. Not your Canva graphics.

And the fastest way to build trust in your community is to be loud, clear, and consistent about who you are and what you do. My mom always taught me that the squeaky wheel gets the grease, and she was absolutely right. Most people have no idea what a death doula is, which means you cannot whisper your way into this work. You have to squeak. Loudly. Proudly. Repeatedly.

I talk about being a death doula everywhere. In person. Online. At the coffee shop. At networking events. If someone sits still long enough, they are going to learn what I do.

And in today's world, one of the most powerful tools you have to spread that message is social media.

Social media is essentially free advertising. It's a platform where you can educate, share your perspective, tell stories, and help people understand what death doulas actually do. And the best part is that you don't have to be famous or have a massive following for it to work. Sometimes the person who needs you most is the one person who sees your post on the exact day they're searching for help.

More and more people are using social media the same way they use Google. They search TikTok, Instagram, YouTube, or Facebook to learn about things they've never encountered before. They type questions like "what happens when someone is dying," "how to prepare for death," or "what does a death doula do." If you are there sharing helpful information, answering questions, and speaking openly about death, you become part of that discovery process.

That visibility matters.

Because most people will never hire a death doula they've never heard of.

When you show up consistently online, you are helping people become familiar with the idea of death doulas long before they ever need one. You're planting seeds. You're normalizing the conversation. You're building trust before the phone ever rings.

And when the day comes that someone's parent is dying or their spouse receives a terminal diagnosis or they realize they want support navigating the end of life, guess who they remember?

The person who has been talking about death in a calm, honest, human way all along.

You.

So use the tools that exist. Speak about your work. Educate your community. Share what you know. The goal is not to chase followers or become an influencer. The goal is to make this work visible so the people who need it can actually find you.

Because you can be the most compassionate, skilled doula in the world, but if no one knows you exist, you cannot help them.

And death work deserves to be seen.

The Business Basics (Without Losing Your Soul)

When I started my doula business, I didn't know a single thing about running. . .well, a business. I came straight out of the nursing world, where HR prints your business cards, scheduling is handled by someone with a clipboard, and nobody expects you to know what Canva is.

I didn't know how to market myself, build a brand, create a contract, invoice anyone, or network. Someone told me once, "You should really start networking," and I had to literally Google "what is networking?" So, if you're reading this and you feel behind, like you're late to the party, like everyone else got a "How to Business" handbook and you got a trauma response and a dream, I see you. You are not broken. You are just new to a world that was never taught to you.

And here's the part I want you to hear clearly: the business side should not be the thing that breaks you before you even get started.

The truth is, you're already doing the emotional and spiritual heavy lifting. You're learning how to sit with fear. How to hold grief without trying to fix it. How to speak about death with love and honesty.

That alone is a lot. If the business side becomes chaotic, you will start to associate your calling with dread. And I don't want that for you.

BEING A DOULA ISN'T "THE JOB," IT'S ONE OF THE JOBS

One of the biggest surprises for new doulas is how much being a business owner entails. You are not "just a doula." You're also the:

- Marketing team
- Admin team
- Finance department
- Scheduling coordinator
- Website designer
- Social media manager
- Intake coordinator
- CEO
- Person holding someone's hand while they die

It's a lot. It can feel like being asked to run a whole hospital unit with one clipboard and a coffee. And that's where so many doulas get stuck or fail to move forward. They fail because they don't build a structure sturdy enough to hold the work.

And death doula work isn't like opening a cute bakery where people walk by and say, "Omg yes, I've been craving croissants." You're offering support around death, the thing people spend their whole life avoiding like it's a haunted house.

That means if you're quiet about it, the clients will not "just find you." They won't, I promise.

So yes, your presence is your marketing. Not in a fake, performative way. In a real way. The way you speak about death matters. The way you explain what you do matters. The way you show up matters.

You're not just building a business. You're building a bridge between death and people who are terrified to even look at it.

YOUR BRAND IS NOT YOUR LOGO, IT'S YOUR NERVOUS SYSTEM

People think branding is fonts and colors. Sure. That helps. But the real brand is what people feel when you speak. Do they feel safe?

Do they feel like you can handle the truth? Do they feel like you'll stay steady when things get hard? That is branding.

You can have the cutest website on Earth, but if your voice shakes every time you say, "I'm a death doula," people will feel that. If you're apologizing for your own existence, clients won't trust you to guide them through the hardest moment of their life.

A lot of new doulas think they have a business problem when, really, they have a confidence problem. They don't struggle with contracts. They struggle with saying what they do out loud like it's a normal sentence. They don't struggle with marketing. They struggle with believing they're allowed to take up space.

And I'm not saying that to be harsh. I'm saying it because I lived it. Confidence is the spark that lights everything else up. Trust in this work starts with the trust you build in yourself.

PRICING: THE PLACE WHERE MOST DOULAS CRUMBLE

Let's talk about pricing because I know this is where many doulas start sweating. Not because you're greedy. Because you're tender-hearted. Because you care. Because you don't want to feel like you're taking advantage of someone in a vulnerable time.

I was terrified to charge people. I undervalued myself constantly. I whispered my prices like I was confessing a crime.

But the truth is, this work is valuable.

Not everyone is built to walk beside death the way we are. Not everyone can sit in the heaviness, the beauty, the chaos, the truth, and hold it with both hands without turning away. That is a gift. And gifts have value. Time has value. Skill has value. Presence has value.

And what you provide is not "just support." It's autonomy. Peace. Education. Advocacy. Companionship. Clarity. Confidence. Emotional safety. Grounding. A feeling of not being alone when everything is changing.

It took one very special client to help me finally see that.

She was with me for eight months, and she poured into me in a way I'll never forget. She told me repeatedly and unapologetically that I was undervaluing myself. She was an educator to her core, even at the end, and she taught me something I still carry:

> *If you don't value your work, nobody else will know how to value it either.*

As she advised, I raised my price for my next client, terrified. They hired me immediately. Then they also told me I was undervaluing myself. That pattern finally woke me up. The people living through this know what it's worth.

Here's a simple way to think about pricing that keeps you grounded: you are not charging for death. You are charging for your time, your skill, your availability, your experience, your emotional labor, your communication, your education, your preparation, and the stability you bring into a room where stability is rare.

If you undercharge, you don't become more noble. You become more exhausted. And exhaustion is where your patience gets thin, your boundaries collapse, and your work starts to feel heavy in a way it's not supposed to.

THE BASICS THAT MAKE YOU LOOK PROFESSIONAL (AND FEEL SANE)

You do not need a fancy tech stack. You need something that works, consistently, and doesn't require you to reinvent your business every week.

Here are the tools that helped me become more organized and more professional, without losing my mind:

Business Need	What to Use	Why It Matters
Scheduling	Calendly, Acuity, or Google Calendar	Stops the back-and-forth texting spiral
Contracts	A clear, simple contract for every client	Protects you, protects them, sets expectations
Payments	Square, Stripe, PayPal	Gets you paid without awkwardness
Invoicing	Square invoices or QuickBooks	Keeps your money clean and trackable
Branding + visuals	Canva	Makes you look legit without a graphic design degree
Communication	A business email + boundaries	Keeps your energy from getting drained by constant access

And let me say something that will save you years of stress: boundaries are not rude. Boundaries are business infrastructure.

For instance, I don't list my personal phone number publicly. I want people to start with email so I can manage my time and my energy. That is not cold. That is smart, sustainable, professional.

Because if you build your business on constant access, you will eventually resent the people you're trying to help. And that's not fair to them or to you.

Doing the (Inner) Work

If I could give new doulas one grounded piece of business advice, it would be this: do the inner work on yourself first.

YOU HAVE TO DO THE INNER WORK OR THE BUSINESS WILL EAT YOU ALIVE

Most of us came from healthcare or corporate environments that taught us terrible habits. Overworking. Ignoring our own needs. Acting like burnout is normal. Chasing self-care only when we're already falling apart.

That mindset will destroy you in this field.

You cannot pour into people at the end of life if you're operating from depletion and martyrdom. You are not here to be a burnt-out saint. You are here to be a grounded, regulated, well-resourced guide.

And here's the truth people don't want to hear but absolutely need to: if you don't build a business structure that supports your nervous system, you will start dreading your phone. You will start resenting your calendar. You will start losing the part of you that loves this work.

Your business should hold you, too.

So yes, learn the tools. Get a contract. Get a scheduling system. Make it easy to pay you. Say your prices out loud without whispering them like you're doing something wrong.

But also, build the kind of business that lets you stay human.

Because the goal isn't just to "have a doula business."

The goal is to have a doula business you can still love five years from now.

Working with Your First Clients

Everyone remembers their first client, but not always for the reasons you'd expect. For some doulas, it's pure nerves. For others, it's panic disguised as confidence. And for some, it's the very real fear that one wrong sentence will somehow cause the entire death doula universe to collapse in on itself.

When I think about my first client, though, fear isn't what comes to mind.

I remember the excitement. I remember relief. I remember thinking, *Oh. Finally, this is it. This is what I've been waiting for.*

That first client wasn't the beginning of my doubt.
She was the beginning of my knowing.

What surprised me most was how easy the *actual* work felt. I had spent so much time hearing other doulas stress about their first client. Worrying they'd forget something important. Say the wrong thing. Sit in the wrong chair. Wear the wrong outfit. Breathe too loud. Not breathe loud enough.

But when you're meant for this work, the core of it flows.

Being present. Listening deeply. Holding space. Grounding families. Offering structure without control. Sitting beside someone at the end of life. That part felt natural, almost instinctive.

Trying to make a Canva graphic, on the other hand? Absolutely humbling.
Taxes? Still offensive.
But sitting at the bedside of a dying person and their family? My nervous system knew exactly what to do.

The hardest part of that first client experience wasn't emotional. It was logistical. We had created the most beautiful death plan.

Thoughtful. Clear. Intentional. A roadmap for her final days. And then her disease did what disease does and threw the whole thing sideways. Watching that plan bump up against reality taught me one of the most important lessons I now teach every single doula I train: **every death plan needs a plan B and a plan C.**

Not because you're doing it wrong. But because death is unpredictable.

Flexibility is not failure. It's wisdom.

The easiest part of that first client relationship surprised me too. It was being the project manager of her entire support system. This woman had a full team around her: two adult children, multiple home care aides, her sister, her best friend, hospice, and me. Lots of people. Lots of opinions. Lots of moving parts. And one of my natural strengths is stepping into that kind of chaos calmly and saying, "Okay. Let's get organized."

I bought a big scheduling book so we could coordinate visits and make sure she was never left alone. I created a communication notebook so everyone caring for her could leave notes for the next person. As her needs changed, I posted simple signs around the house, so people knew where things were and how to help without constantly asking. When her condition shifted, I gathered everyone together and re-educated the entire team, so we stayed aligned.

It wasn't stressful. It felt like breathing. Like this was exactly what I was built to do.

And there were moments, many moments, where I felt that deep internal click of *this is right*. The way her face softened when she saw me walk in. The way her family leaned into the support. The ease that settled into the room when I arrived. Those are the moments death doulas live for, especially in the beginning.

Here's the truth most people don't say out loud: doulas don't fix things. We support. And even imperfect support is infinitely better than no support at all.

Your first client does not need you to be a superstar. They need you to be steady. Present. Kind. Honest. Grounded. Willing to walk beside them without trying to lead the parade.

Everything else comes with time.

During those first client relationships, focus on what actually matters:

- **Presence.** Truly being there, not just physically, but emotionally.
- **Listening.** Beyond the words, beyond the surface, beyond your own anxiety.
- **Attunement.** Every family is different emotionally, culturally, spiritually, and logistically.
- **Education.** You'll offer it, but you'll receive just as much.
- **Comfort and grounding.** You are the calm in the storm, even when the storm is loud.
- **Adaptability.** Plans shift. Energy shifts. Needs shift. You will too.

And yes, new doulas make mistakes. Not because they're careless, but because this work is layered, emotional, and deeply human. Some doulas over-explain because silence feels scary. Some overstep because they care so deeply and want to fix everything. Some forget their own boundaries and drown in the emotional tide. Some get swallowed by family dynamics. Some avoid hard conversations because they don't want to upset anyone.

But here's the thing about avoiding hard conversations: things don't get easier. They get messier.

As doulas, we cannot shy away from talking about the logistics of dying. Advance directives. Body care. Wishes. The practical steps that protect autonomy. These are not morbid conversations. They are grounding ones. By the time someone hires a death doula, they already know where their story is headed. Helping them plan isn't scary. It's comforting. It gives people power, clarity, and relief.

When I look back on what made that first client experience beautiful, it wasn't perfection. It wasn't flawless execution. It was the relationship. The trust that grew between me and a family who had let me into the most intimate moment of their lives. The softness of the room. The connection. The mutual learning.

And if there's one thing I want doulas to understand about those early clients, it's this: you are not the only one doing the helping.

They are shaping you, too.

Every client will teach you something. Every family will stretch your skills. Every death will strengthen your intuition and deepen your confidence. I have yet to meet a doula who said, "I helped someone labor out of life, and it was meaningless." Even when the death is complicated. Even when things don't go according to plan. Even when it's messy. The act of walking someone across that threshold is always profound.

Your first client isn't just the start of your work.

It's the beginning of the version of you this work has been calling forward all along.

CHAPTER 13

The Future of Death Work

The Evolving Role of the Death Doula

The energy around death is changing; people are finally turning *toward* death instead of running from it, and it's honestly fascinating to witness.

Something changed, shifted, and cracked open.

We are raising generations of people who will not be terrified of the last chapter of their lives. We're teaching people how to plan, how to advocate, how to comfort, how to choose, how to say goodbye, and how to live fully while they're still here.

And when people learn about death long before they need a doula, something profound happens. Their priorities shift. Their gratitude deepens. They stop wasting time. They start paying attention. They love harder. They let go of bullshit faster. They live with their eyes open.

The message people cling to is simple but radical:

You can have autonomy over your death.
You can steer the wheel in your final chapter.
And you deserve a death that reflects the life you lived.

If I could redesign education from the ground up, death would be taught the same way we teach birth, marriage, parenting, and money.

Because death isn't a medical failure. It's a life completion. And it deserves care, intention, and preparation.

If you really want to know where this field is heading, picture this: a world where death doulas aren't considered fringe or "alternative" or something people stumble across after 20 hours on TikTok and an existential spiral. A world where death doulas are standard. Expected. Normal. Just as much a part of end-of-life care as the oxygen tank, the hospice team, and all the quiet logistics that show up when death becomes real.

That's the future I see.

I see doulas woven into the fabric of end-of-life care in a way that feels obvious once you experience it. Not flashy. Not performative. Just. . .right. I see them in hospitals and long-term care facilities, in oncology units and pediatric wings, in memory care, in rural communities and major cities. I see them walking into homes where people have never heard the word *doula*, but instantly understand the role once they feel the support. The kind of support that makes families say, "Oh. This is what we were missing."

But here's the part that matters most to me: I don't see death doulas being absorbed into the traditional healthcare system. I don't see us becoming another checkbox role buried under corporate policies, productivity quotas, and insurance billing codes. Because if that happens, we lose the very thing that makes this work effective. We lose our humanity. We lose our flexibility. We lose our ability to respond to what's happening in the room instead of what the chart says should be happening.

What I see instead is partnership, not employment. Collaboration, not hierarchy.

I see doulas running their own businesses, holding their own autonomy, and walking into hospitals, hospices, and care teams as respected equals. Not as volunteers. Not as "extras." Not as emotional support mascots. But as professionals with a clearly defined role in the care continuum. Because let's be honest: healthcare is drowning. Burnout is everywhere. Nurses are stretched thin. Physicians are overloaded. Social workers are carrying impossible caseloads. Patients and families are overwhelmed and scared. And no amount of clinical excellence can replace time, presence, and emotional bandwidth.

We walk in with education, presence, planning, advocacy, emotional support, legacy work, bedside vigilance, and the kind of grounded humanity that simply doesn't fit inside a medical chart. We see the person, not just the diagnosis. We see the family system, not just the primary caregiver. We notice the fear behind the questions, the grief hiding under the anger, the silence that means someone doesn't know how to ask for help.

We help families understand what's happening, what's normal, what matters, and what doesn't. We help them slow down enough to make intentional decisions instead of reactive ones. We help them prepare emotionally, practically, and relationally for what's coming, not just medically. And we stay. We don't disappear when the hard parts start.

I wish every dying person had access to a death doula. Because I've seen the difference it makes. I've watched families move from chaos and fear into calm and connection. I've witnessed deaths that were so intentional, so supported, so deeply human that family members later told me it changed the way they live their lives. Most people will never forget the moment their loved one dies. Doulas help make that moment one of gentleness instead of trauma.

When collaboration with hospice and medical teams works the way it's supposed to, it's incredible.

One of my favorite memories was with a client whose death plan didn't unfold the way we had hoped. Her decline was unpredictable, sudden, and messy. The kind of situation that reminds you no amount of planning can control everything. But what stood out wasn't the chaos. It was the coordination. Me, hospice, home aides, her kids—everyone adapted in real time. We communicated clearly and honored her wishes as best we could. It felt like a beautifully coordinated dance, even though none of us had time to rehearse.

This is the future I see: doulas at the bedside of not just some people but most people. Doulas being the first call families make when fear creeps in, when a terminal diagnosis lands, or when they suddenly realize how little they understand about dying. Doulas helping people connect with hospice earlier, advocate sooner, and shape their final chapter with intention instead of scrambling through the last days.

Because right now, most families don't know what they don't know.

There's a study published on PubMed titled "Experiences of engaging a death doula: qualitative interviews with bereaved family members."[1] Families who worked with death doulas reported feeling overwhelmingly more supported, more empowered, and more confident navigating death. Many described the experience as something that changed the way they understood dying entirely, and several spoke about wanting to "pay it forward" by increasing death literacy in their own communities. The relationships formed had what researchers described as a "lasting, resonant effect." That's not just my lived experience. That's data.

This field is only going to grow. And that brings me to you, the person reading this.

The future of this field is sitting in your hands. Every conversation you normalize. Every family you support. Every moment you show up grounded instead of rushed. You are shaping the culture of deathcare in real time. This work needs your voice, your boundaries, your perspective, your courage, and your humanity.

We're not just supporting individual deaths.

We're shifting how society understands dying.

And the world is already different because we're here.

The Shifts Coming in End-of-Life Care

You can feel it the moment you walk into a home where someone is dying.

The air is different now.

[1] Rawlings, Deb, Kristine Van Dinther, Lauren Miller-Lewis, Jenifer Tieman, and Kate Swetenham. "Experiences of Engaging a Death Doula: Qualitative Interviews with Bereaved Family Members." *Palliative Care and Social Practice* 17 (January 1, 2023): 26323524231207112. https://doi.org/10.1177/26323524231207112.

Families aren't whispering the way they used to, like they're afraid of saying the wrong thing or breaking some invisible rule. They aren't sitting on the edge of the couch waiting for instructions from whichever nurse happens to walk through the door that day. They're watching. They're listening. They're asking better questions. They're Googling words they never thought they'd need to know. They're realizing, often for the first time, that they're allowed to be part of this.

People are waking up to the fact that the deathcare system, as it's existed for decades, doesn't always meet the needs of real humans with real emotions and real families. They're starting to understand that just because something is "standard" doesn't mean it's sufficient. They're realizing they have choices. They're allowed to want more. They're allowed to say, "This doesn't feel right," and look for something that feels better.

Hospice is shifting too. More programs are integrating music therapy, massage, Reiki, legacy work. Some are partnering with death doulas instead of seeing us as a threat. Funeral homes are pulling back the curtain on an industry that used to thrive on mystery and silence, offering aquamation, natural burial, green options, human composting. Things that were once labeled "alternative" are now being described as thoughtful. Intentional. Even beautiful.

And alongside all of that, doulas are rising into the places that have been waiting for us for a long time. Where families are drowning in fear with no one to sit in it with them. Where people don't know what questions to ask until it's already chaotic. Where nothing is technically "wrong," but everything feels like it's unraveling.

If I could snap my fingers and change one thing right now, it wouldn't be policy or funding or infrastructure. It would be mindset. This quiet belief that death is something you don't talk about until it's unavoidable. That planning somehow causes death instead of easing it. That acknowledging what's coming makes it worse.

If people understood, from childhood, that death is universal, inevitable, and deeply human, everything would shift. Conversations would come easier. Care would be better. Planning wouldn't feel taboo. And no one would die in fear simply because no one would be dying in the dark.

A Glimpse into the Future

I want to end with a glimpse of what this new era of death care looks like, because I've seen it. More than once.

There was a woman, let's call her Marian.

In another time, her death would have been rushed, confusing, and chaotic. Family members scattered emotionally. Hospice doing their best inside tight time constraints. A death that "just happened" one night, leaving everyone stunned and unsure.

But Marian didn't die in the old era.

Her family brought me in months before her final decline. We talked openly about what she wanted her last chapter to feel like. She wanted sunlight in the room. She wanted her daughter to rub lotion on her hands every morning. She wanted her son to read her the same poem he loved as a child. She wanted lavender in the air. She wanted honesty without sugarcoating. And above all, she wanted peace.

When she began laboring out, the room changed.

Her hospice nurse walked in and visibly relaxed when she saw me. Her children recognized the changes because they'd already been taught what to expect. They knew what to do. They knew how to comfort her. They knew how to comfort each other.

There was no panic. No frantic guessing. No whispering in corners.

Marian died with sunlight on her face, her daughter's hands on her skin, her son's voice steady as he read. Her breath slowed in a room filled with presence instead of fear.

Afterward, her daughter hugged me and said, "This is what the world should feel like when someone dies."

She was right.

And this is what the world *will* feel like, because doulas are helping to build it. We're not just filling gaps. We're reshaping the landscape. We're changing how people think about death, how they experience dying, and how they live afterward.

The Next Generation of Death Doulas

When I picture someone finishing this book, closing the last page, and just sitting there for a second before the world rushes back in, I imagine a very specific feeling settling in. Not exactly excitement or fear, but something quieter and deeper. A sense of recognition. Like something inside them has been gently tapped awake.

If that's happening to you right now, I want you to hear this clearly: that matters.

I want you to feel purpose humming under your skin. Not loud, not performative, not "I've got this all figured out" confidence. I want the kind that settles into your bones. The kind that whispers, "I belong here. I'm meant for this. And the world needs what I carry."

Because the truth is, death doulas are not just participating in the evolution of deathcare. We are the evolution. Every new doula stepping into this work becomes part of a movement that is actively reshaping how people experience dying. Not in theory. In real homes. With real families. In moments that are raw, tender, complicated, and profoundly human.

If you're new to this world, you probably feel some fear mixed in with that calling. That's normal.

There's the fear of not knowing enough.
The fear of messing something up.
The fear of being too new, too quiet, too different.
The fear of standing out. . .or standing alone.

Here's the thing I wish someone had told me at the very beginning: you can be brand new and still be deeply powerful in this role. You do not need to know everything to make a meaningful impact. This work will shape you as much as you shape it. Every client you meet will refine you. Every vigil you sit will grow you. Every moment of doubt will eventually become something you look back on and think, "Thank God I didn't quit."

But there's something else I need to say here, clearly and responsibly.

This book is a guide.
It is not training.

It is meant to orient you to the heart, the reality, and the depth of death work. It is meant to help you understand the emotional landscapes, the ethical weight, the beauty, the difficulty, and the responsibility that comes with walking people through the end of life. What it does not do, and should not do, is replace proper education and preparation.

Feeling called to this work is powerful.
Stepping into it without training is not.

If you're reading this and realizing, "I think I might be one of the next generation of doulas," the most loving thing you can do for yourself and for future clients is to get trained. Not just anywhere. Thoughtfully. Thoroughly. In a way that prepares you for the real work, not just the idea of it.

Death Doula School

In creating Death Doula School, I built the program I wish had existed when I was starting out. One that goes far beyond a surface-level overview of what a death doula does. One that teaches you about death itself, not just the role a doula plays within it. One that prepares you for what actually happens in homes, in hospitals, in long-term care facilities, and at the bedside. One that doesn't shy away from the hard parts, the medical realities, the family dynamics, the boundaries, the burnout, the grief, the ethical questions, the pets, the children, the silence, the mess.

Death Doula School is comprehensive by design. It covers hospice, the dying process, active dying, after-death care, medical aid in dying (MAiD), voluntary stopping of eating and drinking (VSED), long-term care, assisted living, home care, advocacy, communication, boundaries, sustainability, and how to build a practice that doesn't break you. It is education rooted in real-world experience, taught by someone who has lived this work and wants you to be able to do it well, safely, and sustainably.

And just as important as the curriculum is the community.

Because no doula should be doing this alone.

That's why I also created the Death Doula Collective. This work can feel isolating if you don't have people who truly understand it. In the collective, you bring your questions, your doubts, your stories, your heartbreaks, your "what the hell do I do next?" moments. You learn alongside others who are walking the same path. You get support, perspective, and reassurance that what you're feeling is normal, even when it's hard.

If you're sitting here wondering whether you're ready, here's what I want you to know:

You don't have to have it all figured out.
You don't have to feel fearless.
You don't have to do this alone.

You are not here by accident.
You are needed.
You are allowed to grow into this work.

If you feel the pull toward deathcare, honor it. And then honor the work itself by preparing for it with intention, humility, and respect. Get educated. Get supported. Get grounded.

And if I could look you in the eyes right now, you, the one holding this book and quietly wondering if this might be your path, this is what I would say:

Death picked you for a reason.
You were built for this long before you ever learned the words "death doula."

Let that truth follow you forward.

Your Place in the Future of This Deathcare

If you're holding this book, it means something about death caught your attention. And that alone matters.

Whatever brought you here, you belong in this conversation.

Because the truth is, the shift happening in deathcare isn't being carried by one role alone. It's not just death doulas or death influencers or funeral industry disruptors. It's nurses asking better questions. Social workers slowing things down. Caregivers refusing to let their loved ones be treated like tasks. Funeral professionals reimagining ritual. Families choosing presence over panic. And everyday people learning how to talk about death without whispering.

This is a collective movement. And it's already underway.

We are standing at the edge of a cultural shift where death is no longer treated like a failure, a secret, or a word we're supposed to tiptoe around. We are pulling it out of the shadows and into the light. Not to sensationalize it. Not to romanticize it. But to humanize it.

And you don't need a title to be part of that.

What I want you to take from this book isn't a sense of urgency or pressure to "do something big." I want you to feel grounded. Steady. Clear. I want you to feel that quiet hum under the surface, the one that says, "Okay. . .I see it now. I can move differently."

Because real change doesn't usually look dramatic. It looks like speaking honestly when others go quiet. It looks like asking better questions. It looks like correcting misinformation instead of letting fear run the room. It looks like saying the word *death* out loud, without flinching.

And yes, fear still shows up. For everyone.

Fear of saying the wrong thing.
Fear of not knowing enough.
Fear of standing out.
Fear of going against the grain.

That fear isn't a stop sign. It's a signal that you're standing somewhere meaningful.

Every conversation you have about death that's rooted in honesty instead of avoidance matters. Every time you choose clarity over euphemisms, you help shift the narrative. Every time you support someone through loss, dying, or planning with compassion instead of fear, you are participating in this evolution.

And if this book has stirred something deeper in you, if it's made you think, "I want to be part of this in a bigger way," then listen to that. That's how movements grow. Not through force. Through resonance.

For some people, that path leads to becoming a death doula. For others, it means changing how they practice medicine, care for families, build services, show up at bedsides, or talk about death in their own homes. All of it counts.

What matters most is this: **death is not a dirty word**. It doesn't need to be hidden, softened into nonsense, or whispered like it might bite us. It's part of life. And when we talk about it openly, we live better, care better, and die better.

Wherever you stand in this work, wherever you're headed next, start today.

Change the narrative in your own corner of the world.

That's how revolutions happen.

Closing Note: You're Still Here

You just read an entire book about death. The real stuff. The uncomfortable stuff. The things people whisper about. The things people avoid. The things people pretend won't happen.

That alone tells me something about you.

It tells me you're curious. Brave. Willing to sit with hard things instead of running from them. Willing to look directly at something most of the world tries to shove into the shadows and say, "Okay. Let's talk about this."

And honestly? I'm proud of you. I know that might sound cheesy, but I mean it. Reading a book like this isn't passive. It asks something of you. It asks you to feel. To reflect. To question the stories you've been told about death, about care, about what matters, and what really doesn't.

So how do you feel right now? Do you feel a little more empowered? A little steadier? A little more grounded in your body?

Did I scare you at least once? If so, that tracks. I get that a lot.
Did something crack open for you that you didn't expect?
Did a sentence stick to your ribs?
Did you find yourself nodding along thinking, "Yeah. . .this. This is it"?

That's the work doing its thing.

If you're reading this thinking, "Okay, I want to learn more. I want training. I want community. I want to do this work or deepen the way I already do it," I've got you. Head on over to www.deathdoulakacie.com or @deathdoulakacie on your social media platform of choice. You can find everything you need there!

If you're curious about becoming a death doula and want real, grounded, no-BS education, that's **Death Doula School.** I'd love to have you there.

If you're already a death doula and craving connection, support, and a place where you don't have to explain yourself, that's the **Death Doula Collective.** You're welcome there too.

So thank you for being here.
Thank you for reading all the way through.
Thank you for not looking away.

Death doesn't have to live in the shadows anymore.
Say the word out loud.
Carry what you've learned.
And live well, because you know how precious this all really is.

I'm glad our paths crossed.
I have a feeling this won't be the last time.
—Kacie

Acknowledgments

First, I want to thank the people who trusted me at the end of their lives. Being invited into someone's final chapter is one of the greatest honors a person can experience, and it is something I never take lightly. Thank you for trusting me to guide you through your most vulnerable and important moments. Every bedside vigil, every story shared, every final breath I had the privilege of witnessing is something I still carry in my heart.

You have taught me more about death, living, love, and courage than I could ever possibly capture in a single book. In many ways, this entire book is simply a reflection of what you taught me. It would not exist without you. Even now, I feel guided by the lessons you left behind.

To the members of the Death Doula Collective, thank you for always being there for me. For listening to me whine when things got hard, for lifting me up when I needed it, and for encouraging me to keep going when I felt like I couldn't. The Collective means more to me than I can ever put into words. What we've built together is something truly special.

To the death doulas across the world who are showing up every day to care for the dying and support families through grief, thank you. Deathcare is changing, and it isn't happening because of one person. There are thousands of death doulas out there educating, advocating, breaking barriers, and helping people face death with more honesty and compassion. Ten or twenty years from now, deathcare will look entirely different because of the work we are all doing together.

To every student who has come through Death Doula School, thank you for trusting me to guide you on this journey and for becoming such an important part of mine. Watching you step into this work with courage, compassion, and determination has been one of the greatest privileges of my life. Deathcare is not easy work. There are moments when it would be much easier to walk away. But you don't. You keep going. You continue showing up for people during the most difficult moments of their lives, and that takes extraordinary strength. Many of you have become dear friends, and I am endlessly proud of the work you are doing in the world.

To the nurses, hospice teams, and palliative care clinicians who are doing this work every day, I see you. I am deeply grateful for you. Healthcare and deathcare belong together like peanut butter and jelly. Once we truly learn how to bridge the gaps and work together, we will transform the way the world experiences death.

To my editor, my publisher, and the people behind the scenes who believed this book was worth bringing into the world, thank you for helping turn an idea into something real. And to the many early supporters who have followed my work for years, encouraged me, and believed in this mission long before this book existed, thank you for walking this path with me.

I also want to thank myself.

Writing a book while raising children, running multiple businesses, supporting families through death, teaching students, creating content, speaking publicly, and somehow still remembering to feed everyone (including the pets) was no small task. There were many moments when this felt overwhelming. But I kept going. I pushed through the doubt, the exhaustion, and the chaos of everyday life. Past Kacie went through a lot to get here. Healthcare put her through the wringer, but it also led her to this exact moment. It led her to the realization that we have to do death differently. This book is part of that promise to keep pushing for change.

To my boys, Jon, David, and Jackson. You are my reason for wanting to be great. You are the reason I want to change the world. I love you more than anything, and being your mom is the most important role I will ever have. Jackson, thank you for helping me see and experience the world differently. You have made me a better person and a better doula.

To my mom, thank you for raising me to be the strong, independent woman I am today, and for listening to me complain about all of it along the way.

To my friends who held me together during moments when I might have otherwise fallen apart, thank you. And a special thank-you to Grace, my sounding board, my unpaid business partner, my unpaid therapist, and one of my greatest friends. I would not have made it through this journey without you.

Finally, to you, the reader. My hope is that this book helps you feel a little less afraid of death and a little more intentional about how you live. Because if there's one thing death has taught me, it's that life is far too precious to sleepwalk through it.

Thank you for being here.
—Kacie

About the Author

Kacie Gikonyo is a registered nurse turned death doula who is dedicated to changing the way we talk, think, and feel about death through education, advocacy, and compassionate end-of-life care.

Kacie graduated from Kent State University and became a registered nurse in 2011. Throughout her nursing career she worked across long-term care, skilled nursing, acute care, and memory care settings, holding a variety of leadership roles including Assistant Director of Nursing, Director of Education, Infection Preventionist, and Unit Manager. Over the years she witnessed the same gaps in end-of-life care again and again. Families were overwhelmed, conversations were avoided, and too many people faced death without the guidance and support they needed.

Working on the frontlines during the COVID-19 pandemic made something extraordinarily clear to her: she was being called to something bigger than traditional healthcare. She realized her work was not just about helping people live but about helping people die with intention, dignity, and support.

Since then, Kacie has sat bedside with hundreds of individuals and families as they navigated the final chapter of life. These experiences became the foundation of her work as a death doula and ultimately inspired this book.

In 2022, Kacie founded Death Doula School, an RN-led training program designed to provide comprehensive, real-world education for those called to support people at the end of life. The program draws on Kacie's clinical background, bedside experience, and the insights of respected leaders in the end-of-life space. Death Doula School focuses on meaningful education, practical skills, and ongoing support so students leave prepared to truly serve their communities.

Since its founding, the school has trained a growing network of death doulas across the United States and around the world.

Kacie is also the founder of the Death Doula Collective, a professional community that provides support, mentorship, and resources for doulas working in the field. Through her work, she is passionate about bridging the gap between healthcare and deathcare and believes that within the next decade it will become standard for hospitals and healthcare systems to integrate death doulas into patient care.

With more than 150,000 followers across social media platforms, Kacie has become a leading voice in modern death education. Her work has been featured in national, international and industry media, including *People Magazine* and *Hospice News*, and she is a sought-after speaker at conferences, hospitals, universities, and healthcare organizations.

Kacie lives in Cleveland, Ohio, with her three boys, who remind her every day why living well matters just as much as dying well.

Through Death Doula School and her public education work, Kacie continues to train and inspire the next generation of death doulas while helping the world approach death with more openness, preparation, and compassion.

Index